The
Healthy Lush

A guilt-free guide to nutritious
drinking and living a lush life

And a bunch of other random
useful information about alcohol

Brooke Peavley

Ann Gardner

This book is dedicated to the rest of our family who is so tired of hearing about the Healthy Lush they all might need a drink!

Special thanks to Kim Davis, Ofek Hayon and Mark Lewis

Cover by Robby Stowe

Table of Contents

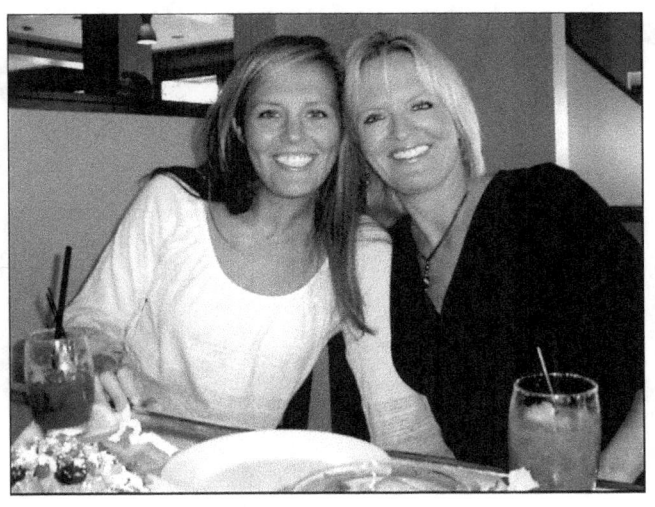

**The fateful day we decided
to write this book...**

About The Authors

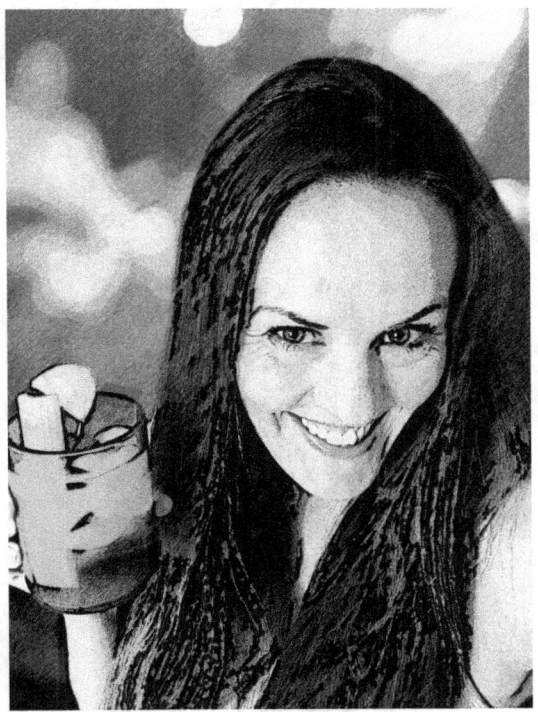

Before we begin, let's explain a little bit about the authors. My name is Brooke, and I'm not a professional lush OR a health care professional of any kind. I'm just a regular girl probably much like yourself, who enjoys an occasional (I'm using the term loosely) drink, BUT who also enjoys living a very active and healthy lifestyle.

My mom, the co-author of this book...well I'm afraid she still needs some work! See those water guns? Well, it's not water! She is at Burning Man, enjoying herself a little too much, and she was happy to have learned all the tricks on how to survive and recover when she got home...

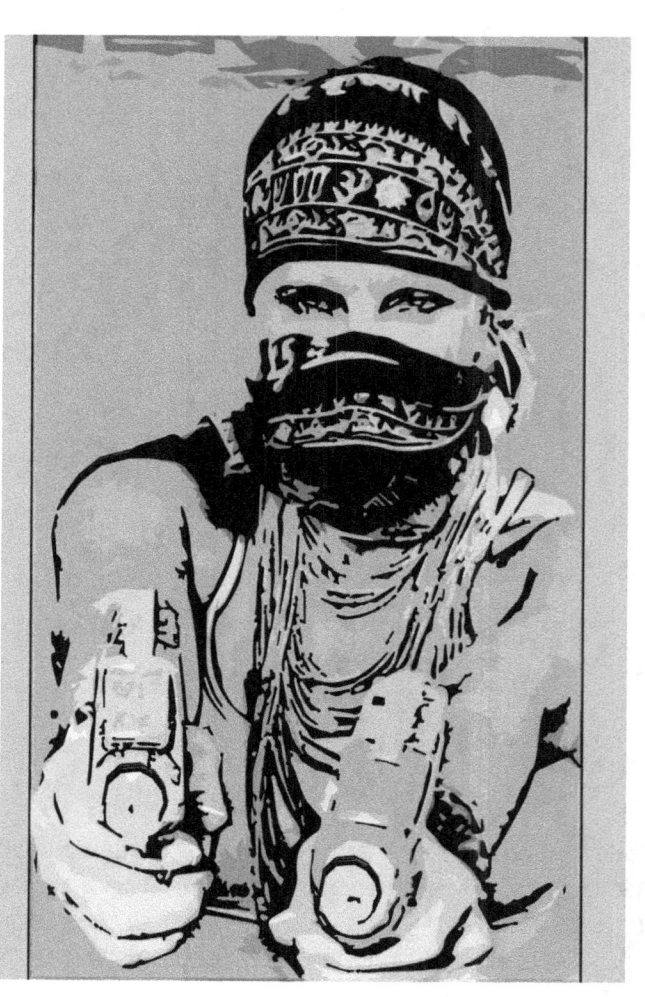

TIPsy

Start drinking BEFORE a broken heart!

My mom loves to have fun and tries to sneak it in whenever possible in our crazy busy worlds. She and I were having a great dinner alone together, finally relieved of any kids, totally enjoying our time and our 'adult beverages' when the subject turned to nutrition... She said; "wouldn't it be awesome if drinking was actually good for you? And we could drink and not feel so damn guilty?" or something like that... We started to talk about how great it would be to know what alcohol actually does to our bodies, how to eat, what vitamins to take or do whatever we needed to offset the negative effects of alcohol. Since nutrition is one of my favorite topics and drinking is one of my mom's favorite pastimes, thus began our quest.

Actually, we both eat healthy, watch our calorie intake, work out regularly, and enjoy yoga and the occasional spin class. We also very much enjoy a night out with girlfriends, and traveling the world to experience a great new alcoholic beverage we hadn't heard of before.

If you're like us, you probably don't want to give up the healthiness of your lifestyle just to enjoy a girls' night out—or in my mom's case, a week out. Fortunately for you, we have discovered through many grueling, focused case studies and hours of research how we can enjoy both the healthy life, and the healthy lush! So my girls (and boys) who are fun, free, and healthy...read on, and enjoy! Oh, and PS. Reading this book will be much more fun with your favorite beverage in hand!

BOTTOMS UP!

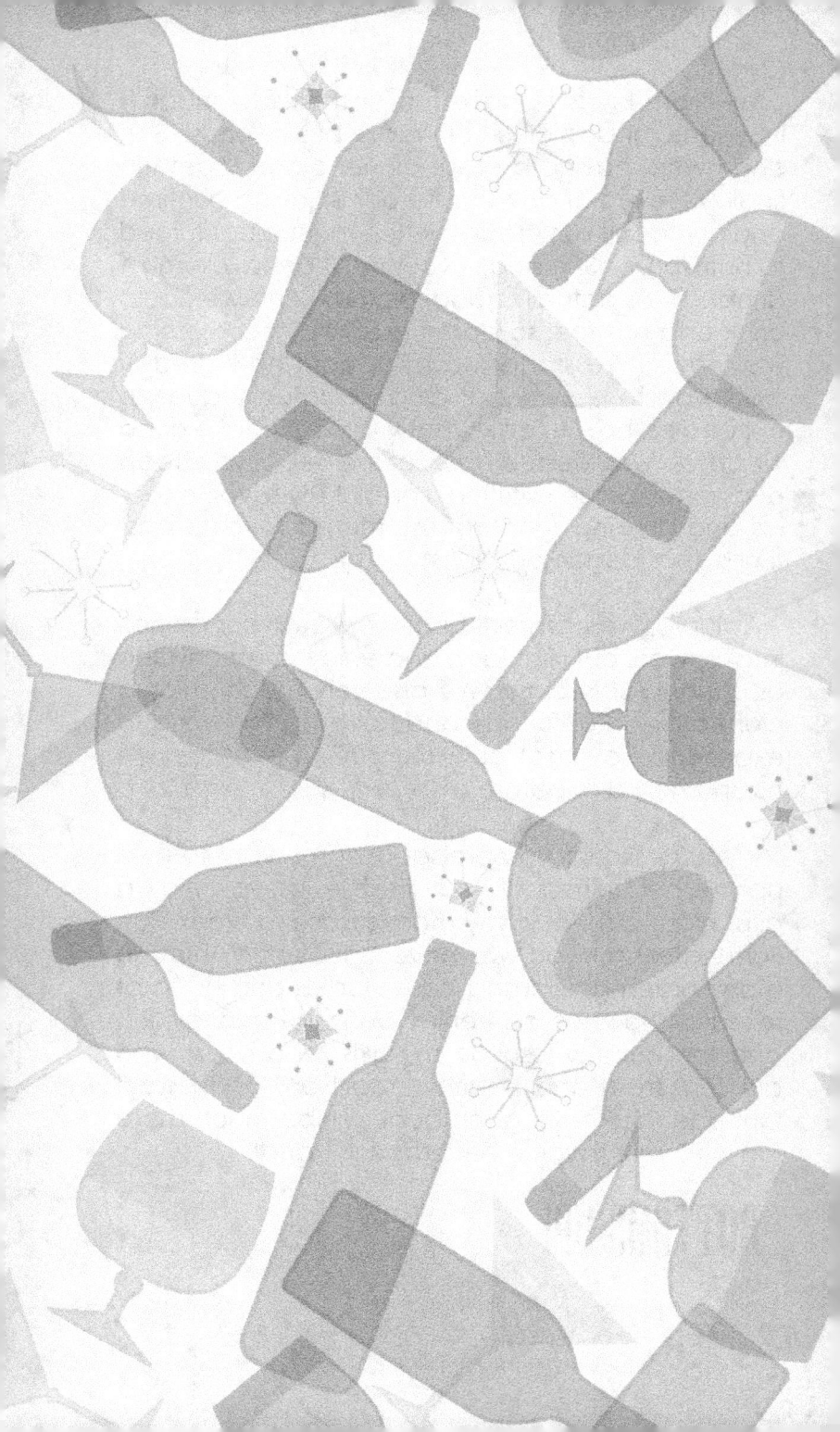

LIVING A HEALTHY AND SOMEWHAT LUSHY LIFE

The purpose of this book is to help you figure out the best way to enjoy the fun and pleasure of drinking, while staying healthy and enjoying life, with a minimum of negative physical consequences. We can't help you with the emotional consequences, though. Sorry!

Every diet, in one way or another, tells you not to drink alcohol. Yet almost sixty percent of Americans consider themselves moderate drinkers, and let's be realistic, these are only the admitted drinkers. The term "moderate," as it relates to alcohol, is defined as one to two drinks per day for women, and two or three drinks per day for men. Right now, after having read that statistic, you're probably thinking, "OMG I hardly drink at all compared to most," or "Yay, I can drink more," or "WTF, I'm checking myself into the Betty Ford Clinic right now." More likely, if you're a really heavy drinker, it just made you open a bottle of wine!

The Healthy Lush

A drink in this context means one 1.5-ounce shot, one 12-ounce beer or one 6-ounce glass of wine. But a word of caution—this does not mean you can add them together for a total of fourteen drinks on Saturday night—unless, of course, it is absolutely necessary!

While drinking in moderation is the standard recommendation, we definitely understand that certain times may arise where you just want to let your hair down.   While there's nothing wrong with letting your hair down, the problem is what else you let down at the same time. Mm–hmm.

The truth is that if you're smart about it, alcohol can actually be a healthy addition to your life. And for all of you health nuts out there who still love to toss a few back every now and again, we wanted to show you how you can STAY healthy, and still have a good time! Living a healthy lifestyle does not necessarily mean you have to give up your favorite drink.

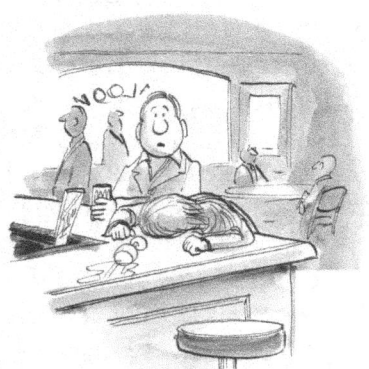

"Tough week or tough life?"

The Healthy Way To Lush It Up

Unquestionably, alcohol used in excess can have severe consequences. Enough said. We know about the consequences of not drinking responsibly. **We're not promoting excessive drinking; we're promoting HEALTHY drinking!**

There's been an extensive amount of research done on this subject...and not just our own. We were shocked to uncover so many positive facts about alcohol, and how it relates to our health.

Let's start with some of the basic positives:

1. One or two alcoholic drinks a day can be anti-inflammatory.

2. Moderate drinkers have been proven to experience dramatically fewer acute hospital visits.

3. Alcohol consumption has been proven to increase happiness, euphoria, and carefree feelings (bet you already knew that!), and alcohol, in moderation, can reduce the risk of poor cognitive performance.

4. Two drinks a day can help reduce the overall risk of cancer.

5. Alcohol, in itself, contains no fat, no cholesterol, and very little sodium.

6. A recent analysis that took data from more than one million people found that women who consumed one drink per day and men who consumed two drinks per day averaged an eighteen percent increased life span than non-drinkers.

A VERY WISE QUOTE
"An alcoholic is anyone we don't like
who drinks more than we do."
(as *Dylan Thomas* almost said)

7. And, most exciting, some recent studies have found that even beer has health benefits.

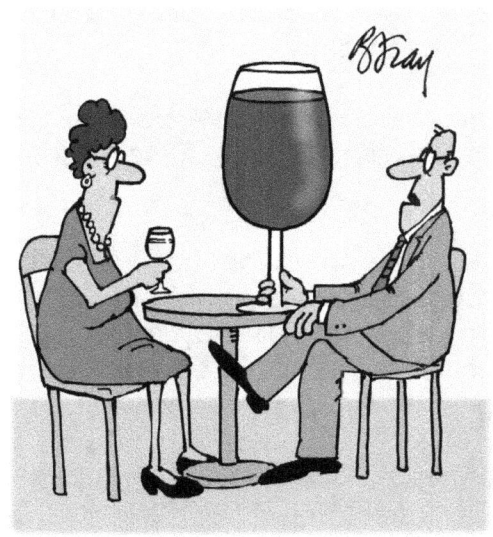

**"I LIMIT MYSELF TO ONE
GLASS OF WINE A DAY."**

A TODDY IN YOUR BODY

Okay, let's be honest. There are only a handful of reasons why a book entitled **The Healthy Lush** would entice you into purchasing it, or picking it up at the bookstore, and inquisitively thumbing through it. First, you're already a lush, and looking for an honest way to become healthier, while staying dedicated to your "lushy" ways. Second, you're already a healthy drinker, and are simply excited to see a "self-titled book." Or, lastly, you bought this book because you know someone who is either healthy or lushy or both, and thought this would be a great book for them to read.

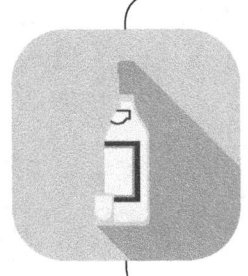

FUN FACT

Alcohol has been used as medicine, religious sacrament, cosmetics, barter, a political tool, bribery, and a generator of tax revenue...

Whatever your reason for reading, as far as we're concerned, your interest in health and drinking makes you an overall FUN human being. We're glad we're enjoying this moment together, albeit miles, and potentially years, apart!

Let's begin with a quick thought that we can ALL agree on—there are few greater pleasures in life than the warm glow and welcome satisfaction expressed by your body as you enjoy a tasty adult beverage. On a scorching day, there's nothing like a cold, crisp beer flowing down your throat to cool and refresh you. On a freezing afternoon, a hot toddy with brandy, or an Irish coffee, brings the blood back to your fingertips, bracing you for your next run down the slopes. Whatever your choice and circumstance, a good drink with fine friends is bound to improve your outlook. And if it doesn't, then it's likely to improve your vision, which will at least momentarily improve your outlook!

We have all seen the studies and read the books about how alcohol (in moderation, of course) can actually be good for you. So, in the spirit of helping our fellow healthy drinkers from all over the world, we have put together a book with some FUN statistics, studies, and facts about HOW YOU CAN DRINK and STAY HEALTHY!

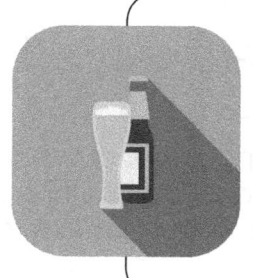

FUN FACT

Consumption of beer in the United States is about thirty-three gallons per person (over age twenty-one), per year.

Heart Healthy

It's not just your social life that benefits from your desire to throw a few back every now and then. There are also many benefits to your heart! Yes, your actual HEART! We're talking about true health benefits here! You've probably heard that a daily glass of red wine is good for your heart. It's true, but it's not the only drink in town when it comes to heart-healthy benefits. In fact, you may not know that red wine is also at the top of the list for the worst hangover potential.

Alcohol's effects on the heart, for both genders, are well documented. Studies have shown drinking a small amount of alcohol daily can raise levels of "good" cholesterol by up to twenty percent, help-ing to prevent blood clots, which keeps the blood flowing smoothly. So the next time someone tells you you've been drinking too much, remind them that it's important that you thin your blood, and do your part to help prevent blood clots.

The effects are similar to what you might see from a low-dose cholesterol medication, or by adding twenty minutes of cardiovascular exercise to your daily routine. However, alcohol consumption alone should never replace prescribed medication or exercise.

Here are some other heart related benefits asso-ciated with alcohol:

1. Alcohol, and other components in alcoholic beverages, reduces the pain of angina, and the risk of heart attack. In fact, moderate

7

alcohol consumption can lower the risk of a heart attack by up to half.

2. Daily alcohol intake reduces plaque buildup in the arteries, and is proven to lower "bad" (LDL) cholesterol.

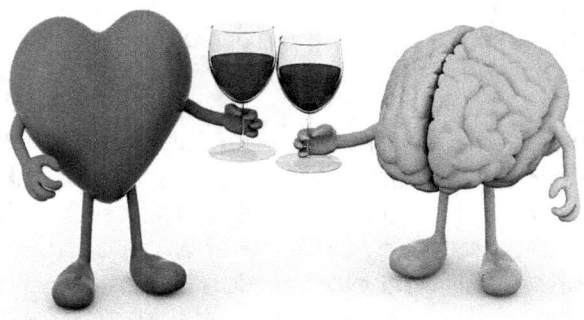

3. Drinking alcohol lowers the incidence of blood clots by inhibiting platelet growth.

4. Alcoholic beverages provide more anti-oxidants than do vitamins C, E, and beta-carotene, and antioxidants help fight atherosclerosis.

5. A Honolulu heart study found a forty-nine percent reduction in heart disease in men who drink in moderation.

Mind Healthy

There is no question that alcohol alters our current state of reality. Remember when you first walked into the bar and realized there were no eligible bachelors in the place, and let's be honest...you did a nice, detailed survey of all the men in the room. Yet after a couple of bottles of wine, the room is filled with David Beckhams. You went from, "OMG, this place sucks!" to planning your wedding and naming your kids, ALL because of alcohol. Ah Alcohol!" We are pretty sure, if there really is over-population, this might be the cause...

BUT alcohol actually has some awesome benefits for your mind, as well as for your body.

Check it out:

1. Moderate drinking can delay the onset of Alzheimer's disease for three years.

2. Light drinking is said to delay dementia and loss of cognition.

3. A diet including fruit, vegetables, fiber, mono-unsaturated fats, and a minor amount of alcohol reduces the risk of stroke.

4. A recent study evaluated the mental abilities of over ten thousand middle-aged women. Researchers found women who drink in moderation had a twenty-three percent reduced risk of mental decline compared to women who didn't drink at all.

Disease Fighting

Most people drink more when they travel. You would think it would be the exact opposite, because "real" life is where all of the problems exist, so theoretically, people should drink more when they're home, and less when they're hundreds of miles away from their issues. This does not seem to be the case, however.

Maybe it's the freedom, the absence of the usual stressors, or maybe it's the hot foreign waiters and waitresses. Whatever the reason, people seem to increase alcohol consumption when they are on vacation, or even when they are just away from home and their usual surroundings.

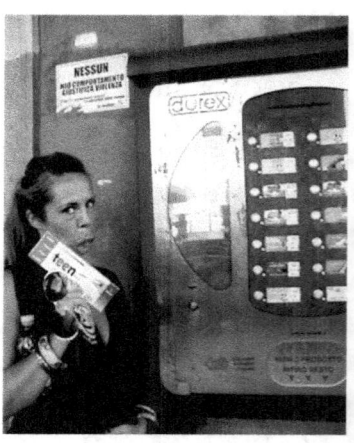

In Italy they have pregnancy tests in vending machines.

One danger of travel is exposure to unfamiliar bacteria, or unexpected illnesses.

Okay, so you can't just pour alcohol over (or into) your body and expect to be "healed," as if it were some evangelical, mystical serum but alcohol can be used as a natural disease fighter, warding off bacteria and things that don't belong!

Take a look:

1. One glass of wine with a meal when traveling effectively fights those nasty virus infections we worry about catching more than some other common over the counter disease-fighting agents

2. Research suggests drinking alcohol reduces the risk of contracting a cold by up to eighty-five percent.

3. Alcohol exerts a protective effect against H. phylori: a bacterium that medical research has determined is the cause of nine out of ten ulcers.

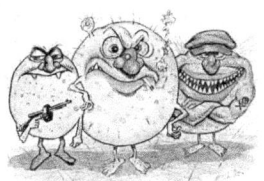

4. Frequent drinkers (those who drink four to six times a week) have a thirty percent less chance of developing gallstones.

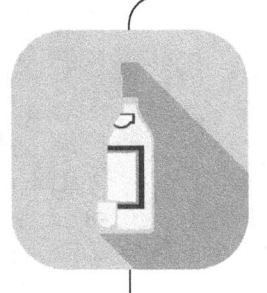

FUN (disgusting) FACT

A popular drink in Cambodia is Tarantula Brandy. The concoction includes rice liquor and - you guessed it - freshly dead tarantulas.

You know what's grosser than that? The Baby Mouse Liquor found in rural Korea. This distilled rice spirit is filled with baby mice carcasses and fermented for a year.

Weight Loss

Wouldn't it be great if this part of the book just said that research has shown that drinking lots of alcohol, any kind you'd like, has proven to cause weight loss? Unfortunately for us, it's wishful thinking. If it were true, we'd be a size two!

However, there are a lot of great diets out there and although they don't include alcohol in their diet plans sometimes its just plain good for the soul to go out and socialize with a few cocktails. It can be a way of bonding and when we are happy, we are usually healthier all the way around. Even those fanatic 'Paleo's' sneak out and throw down a few. If you are watching your weight and want to keep those muscles strong just make sure you are drinking as gluten free as possible. Organic Tequila, Mezcal, and Gin's can be a good choice. Some 'Paleo's' feel they metabolize alcohol better and have less hangover's than they used to... probably because of the high amount of protein in their diet and eliminating so many other toxic foods from their bodies... and we can't say enough about a good workout routine.

For now, let's just say that assuming your alcohol choices are made in a health conscious state of mind, you can enjoy a drink or two while trying to manage your figure. It's all about making sensible beverage choices, and balancing them with a healthy lifestyle.

Here are some facts:

1. Alcohol itself contains few calories, and drinking alcohol does not necessarily lead to weight gain. When polled, women who drank reported a slight reduction in weight compared to women who did not drink at all.

2. Alcohol appears to increase your metabolic rate, causing the body to burn more calories rather than store them as fat.

3. Higher bone density is found among people who consume twelve drinks per week. Denser bones might not sound like weight loss, but women and men with strong bone density have more productive workouts, which produce more muscle mass, and a corresponding loss of fat.

4. Research suggests drinking can increase insulin sensitivity. This has been shown to prevent the risk of diabetes in moderate-drinking adults.

5. When alcohol was substituted for ten percent of normal food consumption in a test, calorie for calorie, all subjects reported a net weight loss.

13

The Healthy Lush

Now you know some of the positive effects that alcohol can have. The next time some expert tells you to cut back on your drinking, or suggests you eliminate it completely, you'll have a few arguments to the contrary. Not that we recommend arguing. Life is too short for that. As a dear friend once told us, "Life is too long to be angry and miserable for the duration." Focus on the positive, and not the negative. Use this book to your advantage. Consider it an educational tool designed to help you reach your goal of making better and healthier choices.

Have a drink, and cheers to the benefits!

TIPsy

A "Beer Belly" is caused by eating too much food. No beer is necessary.

FREQUENTLY ASKED QUESTIONS

Q. Why does alcohol make me throw up?

Basically, throwing up is your body's way of calling you a dipshit. It's saying, you're a freaking idiot—you knew you were drunk five drinks ago, but you just kept 'em coming?

The truth is that vomiting occurs because alcohol irritates the lining of the stomach. The more you drink, the more irritated the stomach becomes, until finally it has had enough. If you already have a sensitive stomach, drinking will irritate it much faster. This is also why some people never seem to barf. They may get just as intoxicated as you do, but it doesn't irritate their stomach as much. Proper eating before, during, and after drinking can help prevent stomach irritation. Another thing that can prevent irritation is not hanging out with anyone who will judge you for throwing up, especially not while you're throwing up!

Q. Why do I pee so much when I drink?

Having to pee constantly while you're sitting at a bar is your body's way of telling you to stop talking to the douche bag sitting next to you...so it's forcing you up out of your chair, and away from the situation.

The Healthy Lush

THAT, and alcohol inhibits the production of an anti-diuretic hormone that keeps your urine concentrated. As a result, your kidneys expel water in your urine instead of reabsorbing it into your body. You will urinate more, and your body will become dehydrated. This is another good reason to drink as much water as you drink alcohol, because as your body's other organs compensate by trying to absorb water.

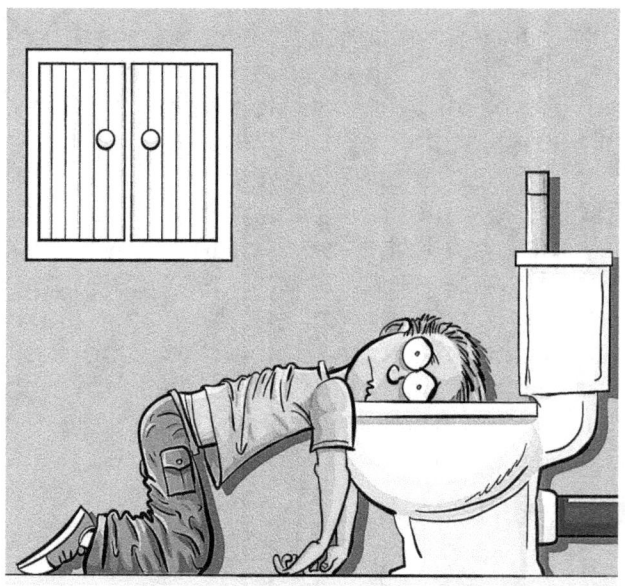

Q. Why do I get so hot when I drink?

You don't actually get hotter. You just think you do. It's called the *"I'm drunk, so I'm suddenly the hottest chick in here"* syndrome, which is completely alcohol-induced. The goal here is to have others around you who are also drinking, so they can share in your momentary fantasy and you're not alone in your delusional thoughts.

The truth, however, is that alcohol actually lowers, rather than raises, body temperature. The heat you feel is an illusion caused by increased dilation of the capillaries, which fill with more warm blood and increase blood flow to the skin, causing sweating, and giving you a flushed look. Be careful! Sweating causes the body to lose heat (and water), and may cause a drop in body temperature.

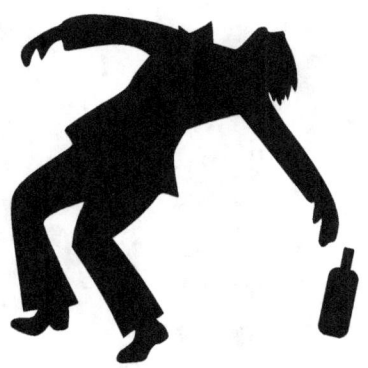

A Very Important Lesson About Water

WATER You Waiting For?

One of the most significant things you can do to combat the negative effects of alcohol is to keep the proportion of water in your system at its proper level. Since our bodies are ninety percent water, we hope you are drinking a bottle of water while you are reading this. You should be keeping the flow going all the time.

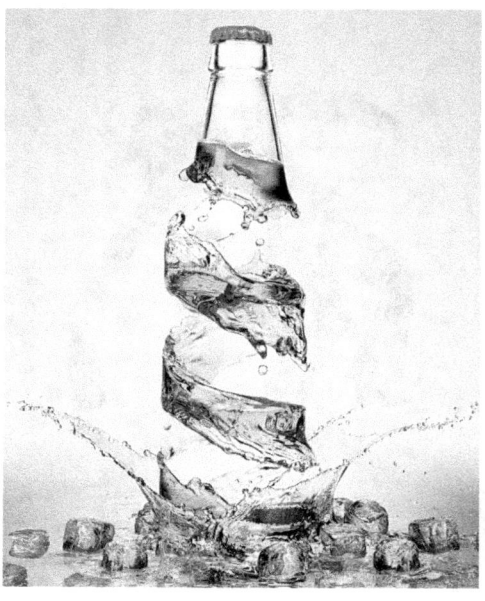

Alcohol displaces the water in your body because it is a diuretic, meaning it causes the body to send more of its water to the kidneys than it normally would. In effect, each beer, or glass of wine, or cocktail you drink is dehydrating you. And don't think just because you're drinking a cocktail that

contains water, that you've done enough to coun-
teract the dehydration process caused by alcohol.
Drinking an adult beverage with a water base in
it, say extra ice, tonic, club soda, or low-sugar fruit
juices, is a better option than no water at all, but far
from the best one.

Sorry to tell you this, but there's no trick to avoiding dehydration. It's got to be a conscious effort.
This is why we cannot stress enough: *AFTER EVERY
SINGLE ALCOHOLIC DRINK, BE SURE TO HYDRATE
WITH AT LEAST TWICE THE AMOUNT OF WATER!* Don't
wait until after the fifth or sixth drink when you begin
to "feel" dehydrated. Start after the very first drink.
The alcohol will mask all your "detection sensors"
from realizing the need for water, so fill up from the
beginning and keep it going.

TIPsy

*Try ordering a club soda with lime after every drink.
It allows you to keep drinking with your friends,
and to quench your body's thirst.*

Besides, drinking a lot of water will not only help
slow down your alcohol consumption, letting you
enjoy more time with your friends, but it will also
give you more opportunities to go to the bathroom
to freshen up, and get away from any annoying
people trying to hit on you.

The Healthy Lush

Another great option, especially on those resort vacations, is pure coconut water! It's high in electrolytes that will help balance your alcohol intake. It's so yummy you'll think you're having a Cocktail!

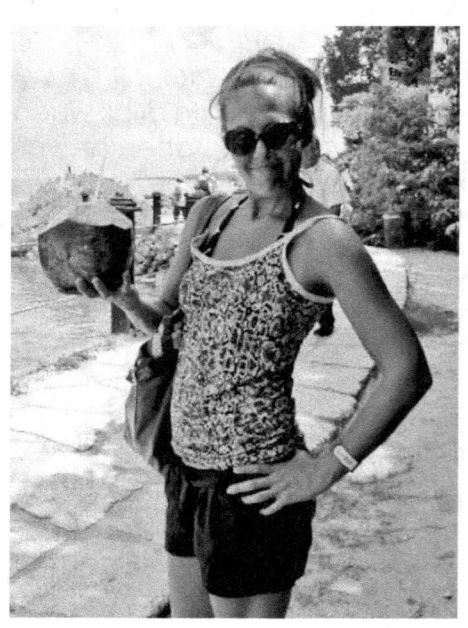

HEALTHY LUSHY TIPS

What's the quote we all know? ***"Beer before liquor, never been sicker. Liquor before beer, have no fear."*** Well, as it turns out, it's actually true.

Here are some quick tips that you should absolutely be following before you consume, while you're consuming, and after you have finished consuming your alcohol!

Do not mix alcohols. Pick your drink of choice for the night, and stick to it. For example, if you're at a wedding where champagne will be served, don't drink a beer first. Stick with champagne, or a glass of white wine, the entire time. Mixing different types of alcohol makes it harder on your body, as your system has to identify and neutralize a wider variety of impurities. When you combine a variety of liquors and then add sugar, you are creating way too many challenges for the liver, and for your blood sugar regulation. Keep your choice in the same family (unless you are the bride or groom!) at this wedding.

Watch your sodium intake. It is best to have your sodium intake balanced (duh!), but this can be tricky—not too much or too little. Stay away from processed foods and additives that spike your sodium levels abnormally. Too much sodium will make you retain water, and you'll feel bloated. If you have only those two choices for mixers—salty or sweet—get salty. Once you're home and it's available to you, take a basic mineral supplement, especially if your food intake has been neglected.

Choose quality over quantity. As with anything else in life, you get what you pay for. Generally speaking, cheaper alcohol has more impurities. There's a reason "well" drinks are always on special. If budget is a concern, it's always better for your health to drink less of the premium version of something, than to drink more of the cheap stuff.

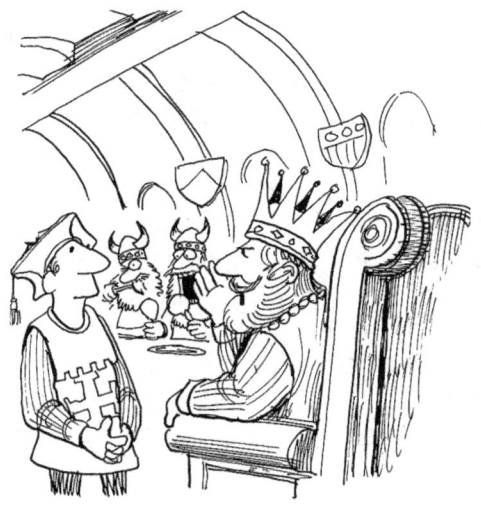

"Serve the cheap stuff, for crying out loud!
They're barbarians!"

Avoid premade mixers. If beer or wine isn't your thing, then you're probably into mixed drinks. Your choice of mixers is a HUGE factor when it comes to making a drink choice. You probably think fruit juice is good, right? Wrong! The fruit juices commonly used by bartenders are usually not natural, and are filled with processed sugar. Stay away from them if you can. If all you have to choose from is fruit juice or a bottled, commercial mixer though, then choose the fruit juice. But remember, alcohol is already causing a spike in your blood sugar, so it will serve you better if you avoid the extra sugar that comes with most mixers.

Better mixer choices are:

- *Club soda*

- *Tonic (diet)*

- *Grapefruit juice*

- *Cranberry juice (diluted with water or extra ice)*

- *Lemon juice (or a fresh squeezed lemon or lime)*

- *Coconut water*

- *Diet colas*

- *Sugar-free substitutes (be careful with these, because too much of that fake stuff will damage your stomach, and could leave you with a headache)*

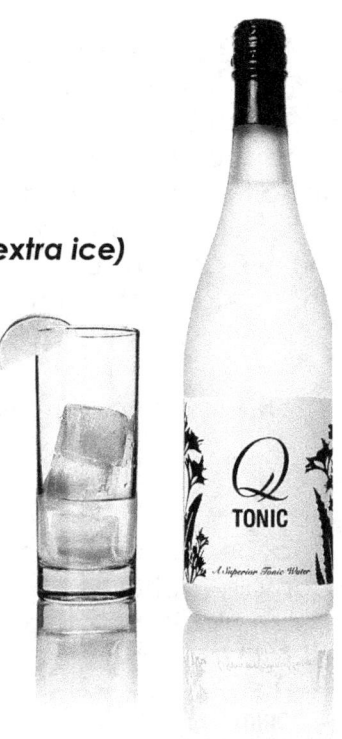

23

TIPsy

When mixing with juice, mix one half soda water with one half juice.

Here's some hardcore fieldwork that we did while writing this book. We talked to several nutritionists to determine what we should be eating IF we were planning on drinking. We were looking for a miracle food that can burn fat while we're sitting on our fat asses. No luck on that quite yet (hurry up, science!), but we actually DID find answers we liked! Turns out there ARE foods that will help you burn a little fat while you're overindulging at the local tavern.

Ten easy foods we recommend, while drinking:

Soybeans (edamame) contain choline, which helps block the absorption of fat. Soy is high in protein and fiber, so it helps satisfy hunger. Edamame is quick and simple to make.

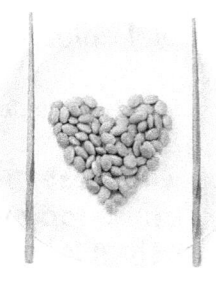

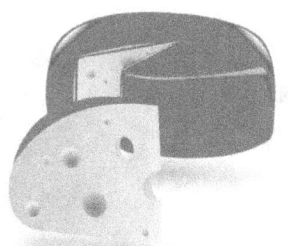

Swiss Cheese is calcium-dense, and can even prevent the release of a certain hormone that causes the body to store fat.

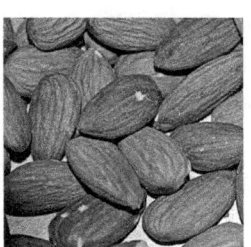

Almonds have a high concentration of linolenic acid, which aids in preventing hunger.

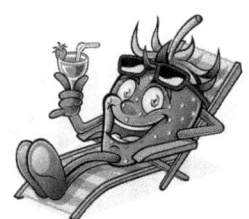

Berries are loaded with fiber and help stabilize blood sugar by preventing insulin spikes. Try them pureed as a cocktail ingredient.

Apples have pectin, which has been proven to lower cholesterol, and they are an excellent source of fiber, not to mention a convenient snack, or cocktail garnish.

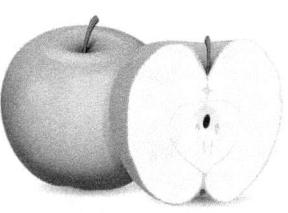

The Healthy Lush

Oranges (and other citrus fruits) contain compounds that help the body metabolize fat more quickly. Fresh squeezed orange or grapefruit juice is an excellent choice for a vodka mixer.

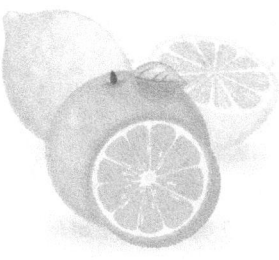

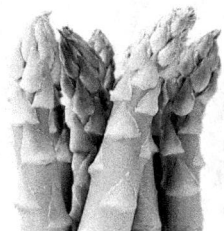

Asparagus contains an enzyme that may reduce, or even help prevent, hangover symptoms like nausea and sweating. Add a few spears to your Bloody Mary.

Eggs have an ideal combination of fat and protein, which slows down digestion, keeping you more satisfied. They also contain Cysteine which breaks down acetalehyde; the toxic substance produced by alcohol. Eggs are a great choice as part of your 'after drinking' meal.

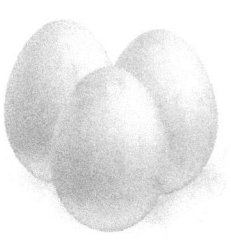

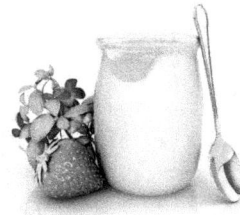

Yogurt naturally contains probiotics, which help in eliminating fat-producing enzymes. Yogurt is also high in calcium and protein and is perfect for dips and sauces.

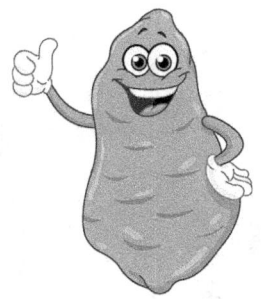

Sweet Potatoes are high in vitamin C and fiber, preventing hunger spikes. Try substituting sweet potatoes as your carb choice at dinner.

Salmon has omega-3 fatty acids with decreasing levels of leptin, a hormone that influences the appetite and metabolism. Salmon is served at about every restaurant, or it's easy to grill on your own.

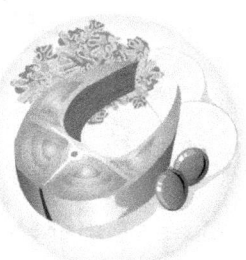

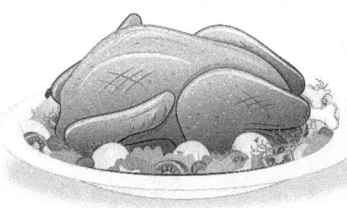

Turkey supplies lots of good lean protein, B vitamins, and amino acids. Also, it's yummy, and there are so many ways to prepare it. Slice it up to snack on later.

And, of course ...

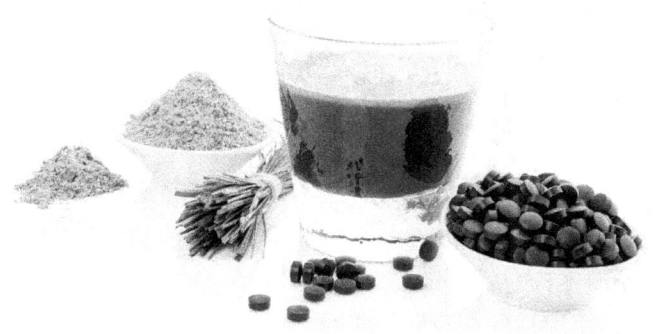

Green Super Foods sprirulina, barley grass, wheat grass, kamut grass, blue-green algae, marine phytoplankton. OK so these may not be the best thing in a martini...but having adequate amounts of these "health heroes" will keep you from over doing the martinis. The best way to get them is in a powdered form or as a supplement.

HOW DRY I AM

May be boring but worth exploring...

Vitamins and Supplements

When drinking alcohol, the MOST important thing is to keep your body in balance. Believe it or not, too much of anything (even a good thing) is not good for you. And yes, we mean anything! In order to achieve this "balance" we talk about, you must be educated about necessary nutrients and chemicals that our bodies need to stay in equilibrium.

There is no shortage of important things your body needs when it comes to maintaining your health. The trick is to ensure that we achieve the optimum healthy balance between things that are important to our physical well being and things that give us joy and pleasure. The problem is when we get together to eat and drink with friends it's super easy to consume too much of what is bad for us and not nearly enough of what is good for us. While eating when drinking is vastly preferable to drinking without eating, let's face it, we are not always eating the kinds of food necessary to get our full dose of essential nutrition. This is where supplements come in handy.

The not-so secret life of B's

B complex vitamins can be the single most significant factor in the impact that alcohol has on your body. A vitamin B-12 supplement is always

The Healthy Lush

recommended before and after drinking. Surely you've heard of the B-12 shots. The rich and famous seem to get them constantly. Well, there are a lot of valid reasons why. B vitamins are the first to go when we drink. While there are several types of B vitamins, we don't want to bore you with all of them. A general B complex supplement will cover all your bases. Understanding vitamins and minerals is very complex. But B-careful. Just because it says it is a B complex vitamin doesn't mean it will actually B absorbed by your system. Choose wisely.

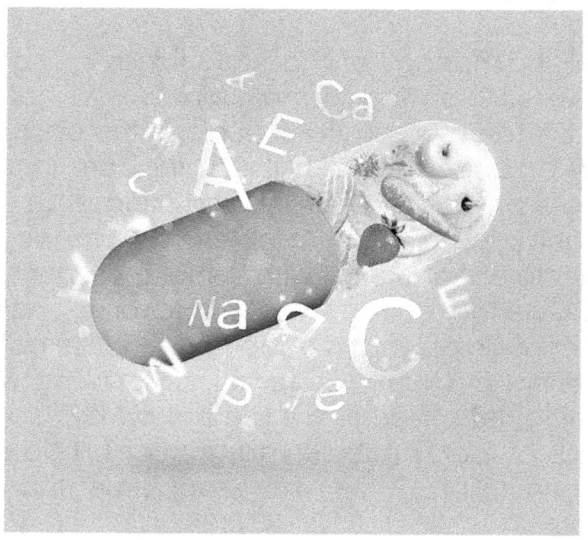

FIBER.... A NEW MOVEMENT

We all know about fiber right? Well, fiber can be especially helpful while you are drinking. It helps fill you up, it helps control the digestive process and it helps flush you out.

Fiber also slows the emptying of your stomach. This is especially beneficial when you drink because it gives your system much more time to absorb the alcohol. Fiber will also help with the sugar imbalances and rises in blood sugar levels caused by drinking. The regulation of blood sugar levels by insoluble fiber (the kind which doesn't dissolve in water...soluble fiber does) helps keep things moving through your digestive system. Nature's Drano.

TIPsy

"No one who follows good nutritional practices will ever become an alcoholic." Roger J. Williams, PhD

Fiber, both soluble and insoluble, can be found in plant based foods such as fruits, vegetables, nuts, grains, soy and some cereals. Products you can put in your water or drink quickly might be an easy way to get fiber when you drink.

Milk Thistle

Silymarin is the main active ingredient in milk thistle. Silymarin is both an anti-inflammatory and antioxidant. Some early research suggests milk thistle may aid people with alcohol-related liver disease.

Green Tea

Studies have shown that people who drink more than 10 cups of green tea per day are less likely to develop liver problems. Green tea also seems to protect the liver from the damaging effects of toxic substances such as alcohol. But how many of us can actually drink 10 cups a green tea a day? Most of us would be buzzing around the office due to all the caffeine but more likely we would just be buzzing back and forth to the bathroom! Start with 1 cup per day and you will still feel the health benefits.

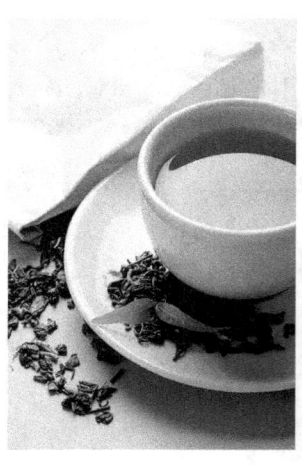

Turmeric

Turmeric has been used in Ayurvedic and Chinese medicine for thousands of years to fight inflammation and joint pain. You know those aches and pains you feel the morning after? Well this might help.

There are many other vitamins and mineral supplements important in offsetting the negative effects of alcohol. Among them are vitamins

C, D, and E, along with minerals such as Boron, Chloride, Chromium, Iron, Magnesium, Phosphorus, Potassium, and Zinc. Again, a vitamin supplement each morning, even when not drinking, is a good thing. There are many out there for repairing some of the damage not just alcohol can cause but just plain old life's stresses... We recommend adding one to your daily routine.

A Few more things...

L-Lysine

Lysine plays many significant roles in the human body. It is crucial for the proper absorption and conservation of calcium in the body. It facilitates the production of enzymes, hormones and antibodies and assists in the formation of muscle protein. Lysine aids in the synthesis of collagen, an important constituent of bones and connective tissues. Besides this, L-lysine benefits involve stimulating the production of creatine, which is responsible for converting fatty acids into energy

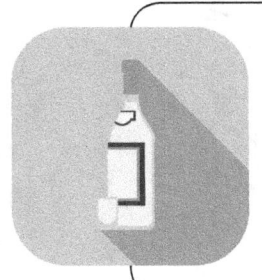

FUN FACT

A world renowned doctor once said, "VITAMINS AND OTHER FOOD SUPPLEMENTS ARE ESSENTIAL for the heavy drinker".

The Healthy Lush

N-Acetyl-L-Cysteine

We found research on this supplement from way back before most of you were born! It has been shown to repair muscle damage... and since alcohol can deteriorate muscle mass, we love this one!

L-Cysteine is an antioxidant. It boosts energy and helps support joints. Cysteine is an amino acid that can be found throughout the body. N-acetyl-L-cysteine (NAC), a modified form of cysteine, has been shown to increase levels of the antioxidants and can reduce cell damage, speed recovery from injury and aid muscle growth. (Yeah!)

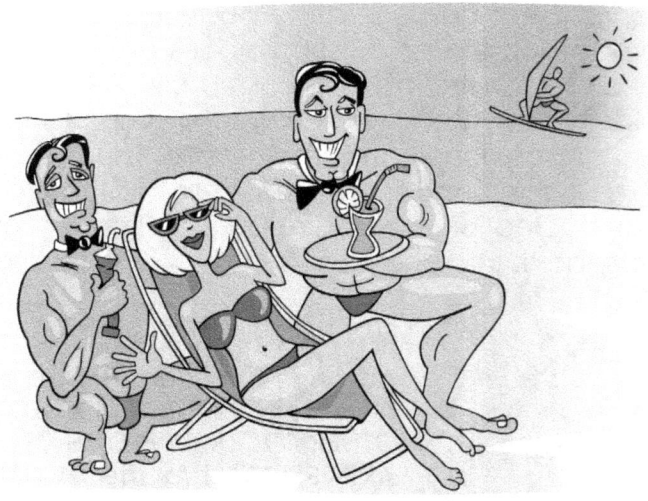

"I just read an article on the dangers of heavy drinking... Scared the shit out of me.
So that's it! After today, no more reading!"

Drinking for your Type?

We don't mean tall, dark and handsome. Eat Right for Your Type has been the pioneer work of Dr Peter D'Adamou and his father in identifying foods and beverages that work better for some depending on their blood type. The proof is in the pudding....many folks have benefited from this food and beverage plan! According to this plan, there are 3 categories: "highly beneficial" which acts like medicine, "neutral" is food that acts like food and "avoid" is food that acts like poison...beware!!!

Blood Type A's do best with a classic vegetation vegan diet. Neutral list: white wine. Avoid list: beer, all distilled, black tea, soda all types, seltzer water.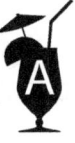

Blood Type O's do best with a higher protein diet. Neutral: red wine, white wine, beer (wheat gluten free). Avoid: coffee (sorry), soda; diet or, tea black.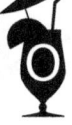

Blood Type B's are classic omnivores. Neutrals: coffee, beer, tea black, red wine Avoid: distilled, seltzer water and all sodas.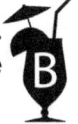

Blood Type AB's need a mixed diet in moderation. Neutral: white wine, beer, seltzer water. Avoid: coffee, soda all types, all types of tea.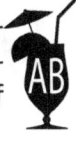

While we have tried this Blood Type diet and do think it has great merit, we invite you to experiment with it on your own.

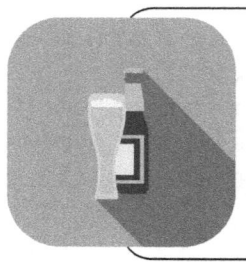

FUN FACT

You know who wins the award for biggest *beer-aholics* in the world?

These guys!

That's the Czech Republic, Germany, and Ireland. SHOCKING, RIGHT? We didn't think so either!

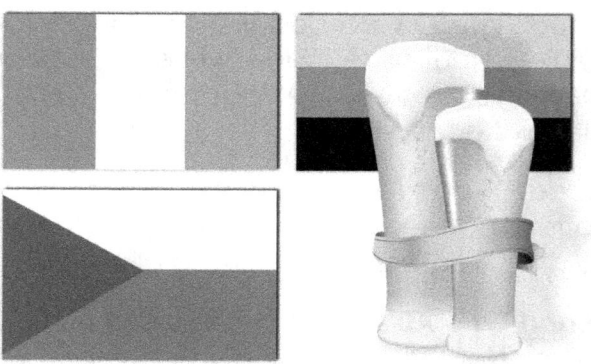

BEER

Seven Bottles Of Beer On the Wall, Seven Bottles Of Beer

The brewing of beer dates all the way back to 5000 BC (that means Before Coors). It was one of the first alcoholic beverages, and the crude process for making beer served as a model for the creation of all other types of alcohol. In fact, in many monasteries the monks were only allowed beer while they were fasting. They perfected the technique. (Now that is our kind of fasting!)

A well-chosen, icy-cold beer can be quite wonderful on a hot summer day!

Here's the skinny on beer.

There are four basic ingredients in beer: malt, water, yeast, and hops. Each of these ingredients plays a distinct and important part when it comes to the look, smell, and taste of the final product.

The Healthy Lush

Because there are so many of you out there who actually enjoy BREWING your own beer, we'll make this section of the book quite detailed, so you'll understand the relationship drinking beer has with staying healthy. There's not much of one.

The malt in beer is grain, usually barley, but other grains such as wheat, rye, or oats are used to make specialty beers. This can make beers high in carbohydrates, at least compared to other alcoholic beverages.

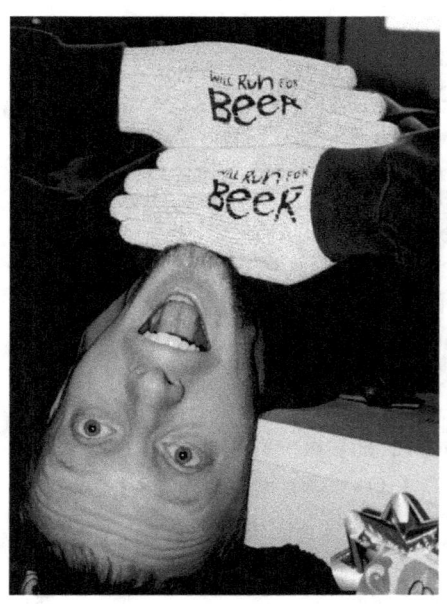

Solely for mathematic purposes, let's say you decide to enjoy three beers with your buddies. If you have three regular beers, you'll have had 459 calories, and 37.8 grams of carbohydrates. If you take the lighter choice (we'll use this for our example, but there are even lighter beers out there), you'll have had 288 calories, and 7.8 grams of carbohy-drates. You've saved 171 calories, and 30 grams of carbs

Over time, that small change will make a huge difference in your waistline.

If you love the taste of a full-bodied beer, then go ahead and enjoy one, but it's best not to make that your drink of choice for an entire day or eve-ning. Think of your beer choice like choosing a food while on a diet. You're going to have to sacrifice something if you want to stay slim. It's that simple.

Since the alcohol content is basically the same whether the beer you're drinking is a light Pilsner or a rich, heavy Porter, the only thing you are sacrific-ing by choosing a lighter option are carbs and cal-ories. And if you just have to have that Chocolate Toffee Black Lager taste, make it the first beer you drink for the night then switch to something lighter. Hopefully by then you'll be buzzed and not care anyway.

TIPsy

In Ireland it's said pregnant women are advised to drink one Guinness a day because of the iron content. You can say you spent the weekend ironing...

The Healthy Choice of Beer

The darker and heavier the beer appears and tastes, the more calories and carbohydrates it contains. The "average" beer contains between 90 and 170 calories per 12-ounce serving. Most beers are fat-free, but they can vary widely in the amount of carbohydrate they contain, anywhere from 2 to 30 grams per 12-ounce serving. The alcohol content of beer is also all over the map. It can range from half a percent (nonalcoholic beer), to twenty-four percent. The average beer contains somewhere between four and five percent alcohol.

These are all obviously wide ranges, so choose your beer based on your overall health objectives, and then based on your personal taste preferences.

What do frat boys, rednecks, and soccer hooligans have in common?

That's right! The number one answer is beer! What they also have in common, all things being equal, is better health than nondrinkers.

Here are just some of the health benefits of beer.

1. Two beers a day for men, and one a day for women, can reduce the risk of strokes and heart disease by as much as twenty percent.

2. Beer increases HDL (the "good" cholesterol).

3. Beer can increase antioxidant levels in your

body, which promotes the transport of oxygen to all areas of the body, including your muscles.

4. Beer contains vitamin B6, which is necessary to create hemoglobin. Among other things, hemoglobin helps maintain proper blood sugar levels.

5. Beer is fat-free.

6. Beer can aid in relaxation.

7. Beer also contains vitamins B and B2 and essential minerals such as potassium, calcium, and phosphorus.

8. Dark beer in some ways is better for you than light beer, as it contains more flavonoids, which are natural antioxidants, which help protect the body from disease.

9. Beer drinking helps reduce the incidence of kidney stones. (And if you've ever known someone who passed a stone...you'll start drinking now!)

10. The carbohydrates in beer are complex, which helps to slow the release of sugars into the body. Complex carbohydrates have many other health benefits.

11. Beer contains water, yeast, and vitamins. This is especially true of unfiltered beer.

12. Recent studies indicate beer helps build bone density. (Don't drink too much, though, or you might end the night looking like you have zero bone density).

13. Some studies suggest beer may be beneficial for postmenopausal women, as some varieties of hops (which are basically little flowers) possess qualities similar to estrogen. You can never go wrong getting a woman flowers!

On the other hand, there are a few things to watch out for with beer.

Sorghum and buckwheat are the most common grains used in Western gluten-free beer.

Here are a couple of gluten-free beers you can find at your health food store:

Dragon's Gold (*Bard's Tale Beer, USA*) A golden amber beer, Dragon's Gold is crafted with pure water, premium sorghum, hops, and yeast, combined with buckwheat, natural honey, corn, and rice.

TIPsy

"Give beer to those who are perishing, wine to those who are in anguish; let them drink and forget their poverty and remember their misery no more."
Proverbs 31:6-7

Redbridge (*Anheuser-Busch, USA*) Redbridge is brewed from sorghum, an old world grain, without mixing or blending, in order to keep its purity.

The carbonation in beer causes faster absorption of other liquids—so any liquor you drink with beer will be absorbed more quickly than normal. This is why beer is the classic chaser after a tequila shot for those younger folks. We know it's very common to have a beer as a chaser for a shot. While we're guilty of this as well, it really is a bad decision. First and foremost, because of the carbonation in beer, you'll become intoxicated more rapidly, and upset your stomach in the process. Secondly, if you are using beer as your chaser that probably means you're not drinking water in between shots. (Two shots should be your maximum, no matter what you're chasing it with.)

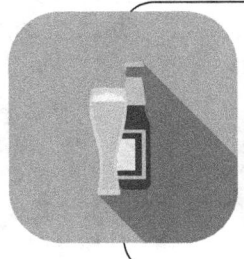

FUN FACT

Russian bar lore says a bite of rough bread with every sip of alcohol prevents a hangover.
(Complex carbs best delay the absorption of alcohol...)

But let's assume we can't convince you otherwise, and beer is the chaser. Do some quick math and figure for every one shot you have, your body will think you've had two. You're more likely to end up with a hangover, and the munchies later on, so don't say we didn't warn you!

- Beer does contain empty calories, and they add up quickly with multiple beers.

- Beer is filling, which can cause you to limit your water intake, leading to dehydration.

- Beer stimulates gastric acid secretion (upsets your stomach), which causes heartburn.

Food Pairings with Beer

"Give us this day our daily bread..." A lot of people think that they shouldn't drink beer, because it will make them fatter than if they drink a mixed drink of some kind. This isn't necessarily the case, as we have seen here. What's important with beer, if you must drink it, is that you pair it with the foods it belongs to. Sometimes pretzels and bar nuts can be just the right thing.

For optimum health, you'll want to balance your diet by eating something other than more bread, or any flour-based product, along with your beer.

Nothing beats cold beer and hot food. Unfortunately, a hot pretzel with your beer is not the best thing you can do. White flour and starches are the enemies here. Someone needs to start making whole-grain pretzels at ball games, right? There are much healthier and tastier choices than salty snacks or hotdogs.

Here are some suggestions!

GOOD

Pizza (yay) is a good choice because of the cheese and other proteins that can be added as toppings. Thin crust and vegetable toppings would be even better, and

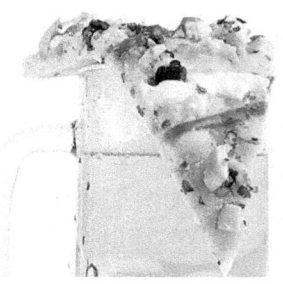

try to get a whole-wheat, or another dense grain, crust. Just remember to stay away from the outer crust edges when you eat your pizza.

BETTER

Mexican food is a better choice, if it is a meal based around cheese, beans, and proteins. Skip the chips and the rice. A corn tortilla is okay, but stay away from anything deep-fried. Load up on beans for the fiber...and for the fun, a few hours later.

BEST

Your best choice to pair with beer is **lean protein**. Chicken, turkey, steak, and fish are all excellent choices. A nice simple salad with vegetables that are rich in color would be a great side dish. At a party, try and hit the vegetable tray, if one is available.

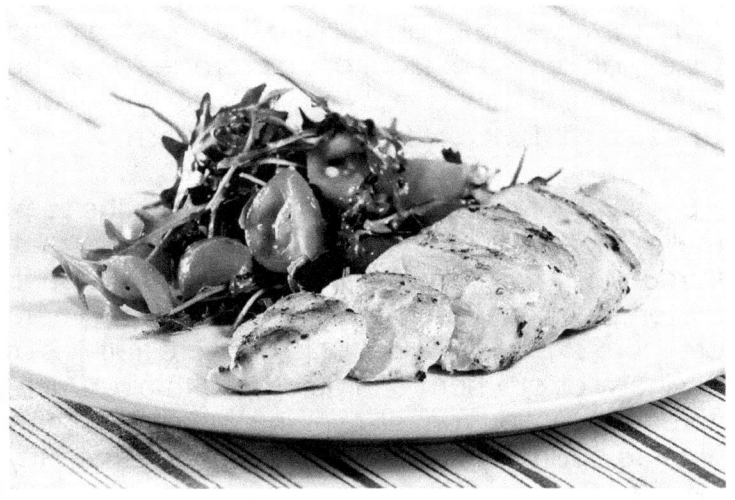

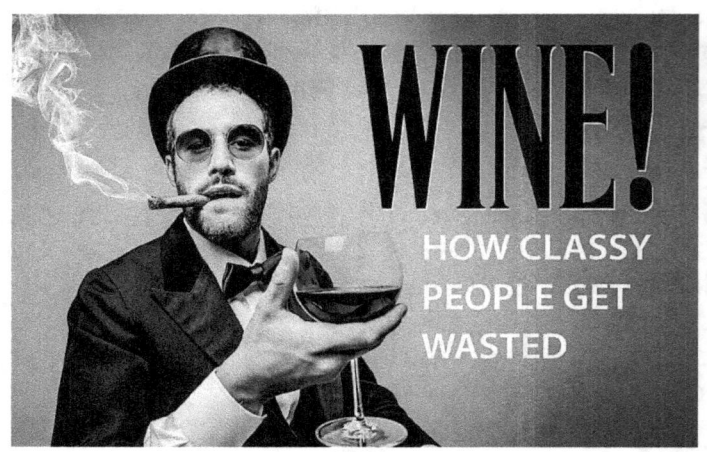

WINE

Some people love it. Some people hate it. But no one denies the popularity of wine. People LOVE to show off their knowledge of wine. Ever seen the movie *Sideways*? There is an entire movie dedicated to wine lovers. There are more things paired with, toasted with, written about, and organized around wine than any other alcoholic beverage. Wine and Dine. Wine Enthusiasts. Wine Tastings. Wine and Cheese. WINE COUNTRY! The list is endless!

Our study of wine is more of a taste from the sommelier's spoon, than a glass of decanted cabernet. If you want to learn more, you can find enough material on wine out there to last a lifetime. There are more experts on wine than there are fruit flies at a winery, all of whom can guide you through vineyards of varieties from all over the world. We simply want to outline how wine fits into an overall healthy lifestyle.

Let's take a little trip through wine country...

What Is Wine?

Good question. The wine the vast majority of people drink is a fermented alcoholic beverage made from grapes. Other fruits, such as berries, peaches, plums, apricots, and so on, are also used to make wine. You may even see wines made from flowers, roots, vegetable, leaves, you-name-it, but these are not wines in the classic sense, as any base ingredient other than fruit requires that sugar be added at some point in the process. Another distant cousin is sake, which is called rice wine, but since it is brewed from a grain, it's not really considered a "wine" for our purposes.

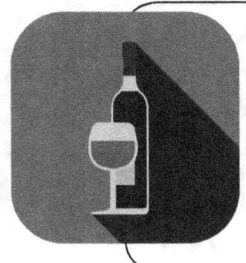

FUN FACT ABOUT WINE

Antioxidants in red wine, called polyphenols, may help protect the lining of blood vessels in your heart.

The fruit sugar (dextrose) from grapes that have been picked, pressed, and then mixed with water, is combined with yeast. This mixture then naturally ferments into alcohol. The resulting juice is placed in barrels for storage. The vessel it is stored in, along with the variety of grape initially used, adds much of the wine's color and flavor, before being bottled and sent to market.

The Healthy Lush

Here's something useful to know about wine: Most of the common varieties of wine are named for the region of the world where they originated. Many of the more recognizable ones were first produced in France: Merlot, Cabernet, Sauvignon, Chardonnay, etc. Cuttings of the most desirable grape vines have been transported around the world, and many countries produce their own grape stock that translates into excellent wines.

Grapes are harvested during the fall at a specific time of day that the winemaker has determined to be the optimum moment, to ensure the correct balance of acid and sugar. They are handpicked, and then cleaned to remove foreign materials, critters, and varmints. Next, they are squeezed to extract the juice.

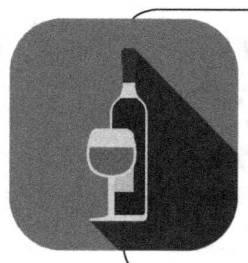

FUN FACT ABOUT WINE
It is a common misconception that all wines improve with age. In fact, more than ninety percent of all wines should be consumed within one year.

Sparkling wine, or Champagne (it can only be labeled as Champagne if it is grown and produced in the Champagne region of France), is made almost the same way as regular wine, with the only difference being the bottling process. During this process sugar and yeast are added and sediment and yeast are removed before corking. A monk (that's right more monks making alcohol! It's a

Godly pursuit) named Dom Perignon created this delightful bubbly drink back in the seventeenth century. He also invented the cork, as it is used today. The special cork stopper is needed because the resulting carbonation would push an ordinary cork out of the bottle.

As with other carbonated beverages, this carbonation also makes sparkling wine intoxicate its drinker faster than regular wine, as it causes the alcohol to be absorbed into the bloodstream more quickly. Other factors aside, and all things being equal, one person sipping on a glass of champagne will become intoxicated faster than another person consuming a glass of still wine.... no wonder champagne is our favorite!

Wine Not

The health benefits of wine are known throughout the world. In Italy, pregnant women are advised to enjoy a glass of wine a day to ensure a healthy pregnancy. On the flip side, it's imperative to enjoy a glass of wine a day to ensure you stay sane while raising children.

It seems every year brings another study attesting to the health benefits of *vino*. Here are a few of the most important revelations.

The Healthy Lush

1. Wine promotes longevity: Wine drinkers have a thirty-four percent lower mortality rate than beer or spirit drinkers. We think that statistic implies that sixty-six percent of winos never die?

2. Wine reduces the risk of heart attacks: Moderate drinkers suffering from high blood pressure are thirty percent less likely to have a heart attack than nondrinkers.

3. Wine lowers the risk of heart disease: Red wine tannins contain procyanidins, which protect against heart disease.[3] Wines from Sardinia and southwest France have more procyanidins than other wines.

4. Wine reduces the risk of type 2 diabetes: Moderate drinkers have thirty percent less risk than nondrinkers of developing type 2 diabetes.

5. Wine lowers the risk of stroke: The possibility of suffering a blood clot related stroke drops by about fifty percent in people who consume moderate amounts of alcohol.

6. Wine cuts the risk of cataracts: Moderate drinkers are thirty-two percent less likely to get cataracts than nondrinkers; those who consume wine are forty-three percent less likely to develop cataracts than those drinking mainly beer.

7. Wine cuts the risk of colon cancer: Moderate consumption of wine (especially red) cuts the

risk of colon cancer by forty-five percent.

8. Wine slows brain decline: Brain function declines at a markedly faster rate in nondrinkers than in moderate drinkers.

9. Wine is loaded with resveratrol: No other alcohol category can claim this. Among the many benefits of resveratrol is that it includes antioxidant properties, which means it is capable of ridding the body of dangerous and harmful free radicals that might eventually lead to the development of cancer. Additionally, resveratrol can be beneficial in protecting the central nervous system, regulating hormones, and can act as a blood-thinning agent.

Of course, it's not all wine and roses. There are some significant drawbacks to drinking wine. (Skip over this part if you REALLY love wine).

When we say drawbacks, we're not referring to when the corkscrew fails, and you have to push what is left of the cork down into the bottle, and then scoop those little cork particles out of your glass with a spoon and...wait...what were we talking about? Oh yeah, the *health* drawbacks to drinking wine.

1. Red wine, and, to a lesser extent, wine in general, is second only to brandy for causing the worst hangovers. This is because wine is served in a fairly natural form, and the congeners (more about these later) have not been removed through distillation.

2. Wine inhibits the body's production of vaso-pressin, which is a chemical that keeps the body from losing water. This can lead to dehydration and headaches.

3. Wine can increase allergy symptoms. In reading medical literature, we found that a few people reported they might be allergic to the grapes in the wine. However, a lot more goes into a bottle of wine than grapes. Sulfites, for example, are commonly blamed for allergies.

TIPsy

So if you feel stuffed up when you drink red wine you might be allergic to grapes (or sulphides)!

Our Favorite...Saké

Although saké is not officially considered wine because it is made from rice, it is still in the wine category. It is actually one of the healthiest alcohol choices. Here are some reasons why...

1. Saké contains no sulfites. Unlike wine, beer, and most other alcohol, saké is sulfite-free. Some people suffer a reaction from sulfites, often resulting in severe headaches. If this sounds like you or someone you know, try premium sake' not only is it delicious but it may be just the cure!

2. Premium Saké can be hangover free. Premium saké contains practically no congeners – the impurities and byproducts of fermentation in alcoholic beverages we talked about that cause hangovers. Premium saké, rice is milled to such a high degree that most congeners are eliminated. In our own experience, when consumed in moderation (wink, wink, nudge, nudge), premium saké is hangover free!

3. Saké has a much lower acidity than wine. Saké has only about 1/3 as much acid as wine, so there's no tendency for reflux and the "sour stomach" one can experience after drinking wine. Easy on the throat and stomach, premium saké goes down nice and smooth.

4. Saké may help prevent diabetes. A professor from the medical department at a prestigious college in Japan found a component in saké that allows fat cells to absorb blood sugar, thus lowering the level of sugar in the blood.

5. Saké promotes healthy skin. Saké contains the most significant amino acids of all alcoholic beverages; Glutamine (creates protein), Alanine (found in

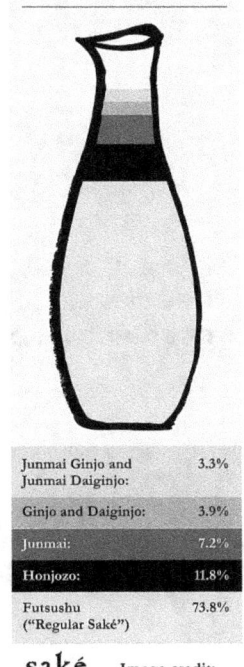

Saké Production by Grade

Junmai Ginjo and Junmai Daiginjo:	3.3%
Ginjo and Daiginjo:	3.9%
Junmai:	7.2%
Honjozo:	11.8%
Futsushu ("Regular Saké")	73.8%

saké nomi Image credit: www.sakenomi.us

collagen), Leucine important for maintaining muscle), and Arginine plays an important role in healing of wounds, removing ammonia from the body, immune function, and the release of hormones. Saké promotes smooth and glowing skin. One Doctor with the Japan Sumo Association clinic has his wrestler's drink saké to promote blood circulation in the skin and as well as circulate and distribute nutrition throughout the body. He even uses saké as a topical treatment to heal the wrestler's skin wounds!

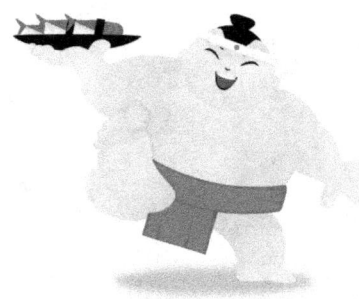

Needless to say... Sumo wrestlers are not the only ones who love Saké!

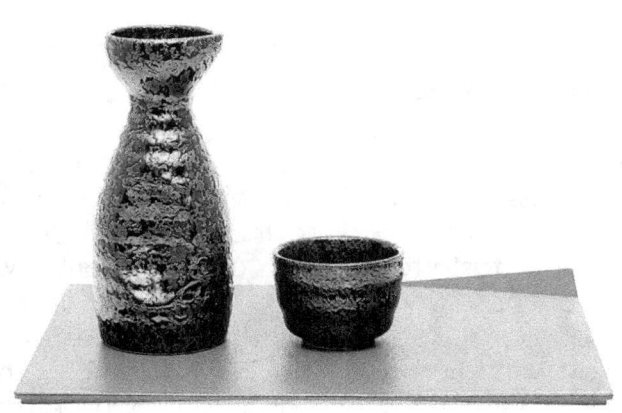

TIPsy

Try a sake bath!
2-3 oz in your bath water can lower
blood pressure and help you sleep...

Food Pairings with Wine

What to eat while you're wining it up!

There are libraries full of books, entire magazines, and endless opinions about which wine goes best with which food. We found that these tend to be a matter of taste rather than one of health. We'll leave your nose and palette out of it, and, instead, give you our suggestions for the healthiest foods to enjoy with your wine. Feel free to use a combination of our suggestions, and your own personal preferences, so that you can still enjoy your wine experience. After all, drinking is never worth it, if it's not going to be a pleasurable experience.

BAD

Sugar and candy—STAY AWAY! Processed sugar will cause a spike in your blood sugar. If you want dessert, go for a creamy one containing protein and/or fat. More and more restaurants, especially nicer ones, and those that have an extensive wine list,

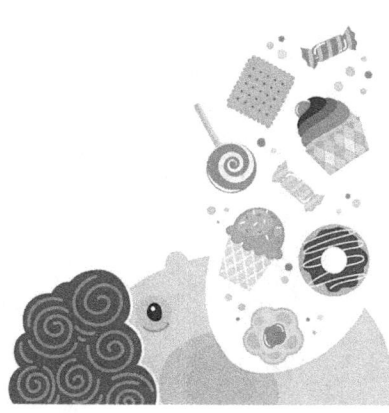

are offering low-sugar desserts. These are a great option to go with wine. You still get to please your taste buds, but avoid the dreaded sugar consequences. Keep in mind that desserts that are advertised as "low-sugar" probably are sweetened with a sugar substitute that your body might reject. Eat sparingly of these artificially sweetened treats until you know how your body might react to them. Don't believe that it's okay to eat these all the time.

Fried foods are another no-no. In fact, fried foods are a no-no whether you're drinking wine or not! They are never healthy, and are especially harmful for your body when accompanied by drinking. As much as we are promoting and emphasizing the health benefits of drinking, the bottom line is that when you drink, you are still putting a foreign substance in your body. Talk about kicking a guy while he's down. Eating fried food while drinking is just like pouring salt into a wound. There's no need to gum up the works even more by forcing your already burdened system to process fried foods. If that is all you are stuck with, a good suggestion would be to peel off the breaded part, and eat just the inside of fried cheese sticks, fried zucchini, jalapeno poppers, etc. So what if you look a little obsessive-compulsive. You will also be the one who looks the best in front of the mirror, and has the healthiest heart.

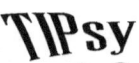

TIPsy

The body and brain are always seeking balance. Remember, alcohol turns into sugar. Nutrient-dense food before the celebration can make or break your next day.

GOOD

Fresh fruit is always a good choice whether you are drinking or not! It adds vitamins and anti-oxidants to the ones you are already getting from the wine. Be careful though because fruit also adds sugar.

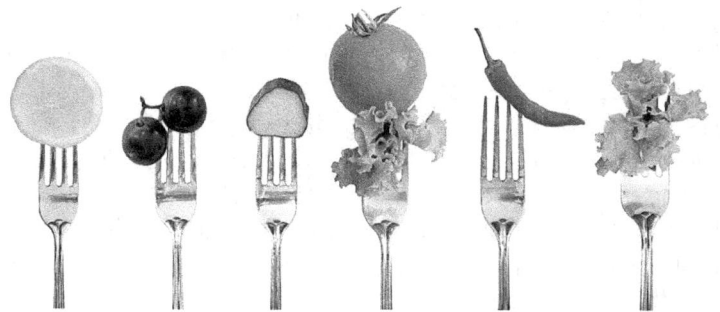

Crackers add fiber to your diet, but they are also loaded with calories, so don't overdo it. Choose crackers made from whole grains to avoid sugar and processed flour.

Cheese is a great source of protein and healthy fat. It also includes amino acids. Like crackers, only eat cheese in moderation, as it is high in calories.

TIPsy

Protein is what's going to help slow down the rise in blood sugar brought on by drinking alcohol.

Bread is fine, but choose a whole grain bread to slow digestion. Rye, seeded, whole wheat, or sprouted wheat breads are some of our favorites.

Pasta is also fine, but, again, look for whole-grain or quinoa varieties, and avoid fat-laden sauces. Sorry 'Fredo. You broke my heart.

BEST

Start with a big salad. A modest portion of dressing will provide a bit of fat to slow down the absorption of wine. If you're dining out, a salad loaded with dark colors, greens and reds especially, is the best way to start your meal. As always, request the dressing on the side, and use a small amount, but don't think you have to skip the dressing altogether.

Soup is another great option at a restaurant. However, not all soup is a positive choice. If it contains any cream at all, then skip it. Soups with a clear or tomato broth are excellent. Try minestrone, Manhattan clam chowder, *pasta e fagioli,* or vegetable chili.

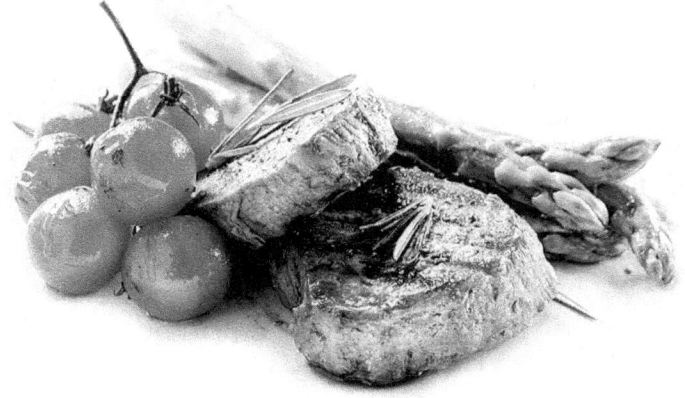

The Healthy Lush

Yogurt is a great source of calcium, protein, and probiotics to help with digestion. It also slows the absorption of alcohol. Yogurt can make a great topping for fish, or, if you sweeten it up, is a perfect dessert to end your meal. Be sure to check the sugar content before you indulge in yogurt though. A lot of yogurts say they have added fruit, which really means fruit-flavored, high-fructose corn syrup, and that's a no-no. Try to pick a plain yogurt or something all-natural.

Figs are an antioxidant. They also help you avoid dehydration by retaining moisture.

Green vegetables are nutritional winners, the more color the better, and have them steamed or sautéed. They provide extra fiber, vitamins, and minerals. Substitute a side of vegetables for the starch of your meal. Think of the starch as you would your wine. That is how your body is going to react. A side of any kind of vegetable is better than mashed potatoes or white rice added with fat. But be sure to avoid decadent sauces or keep them on the side. Vegetables will soak up anything they are cooked in.

Animal protein, especially lean cuts of beef, chicken, lamb, and pork, are a great choice. This should be easy since most wine drinkers are enjoying the grape along with a meal. The great thing about wine is that it can be paired and enjoyed with so many types of meat. As long as you've made other smart choices about your meal, then splurge on your main course. If that means a nice juicy rib-eye steak, then so be it.

BESTEST

Seafood is probably our number one recommendation for wine pairing. There are so many kinds of seafood to choose from, all of which are an excellent source of protein and antioxidants. Excellent choices include broiled lobster or crab, grilled salmon, or swordfish. The options are endless when it comes to seafood!

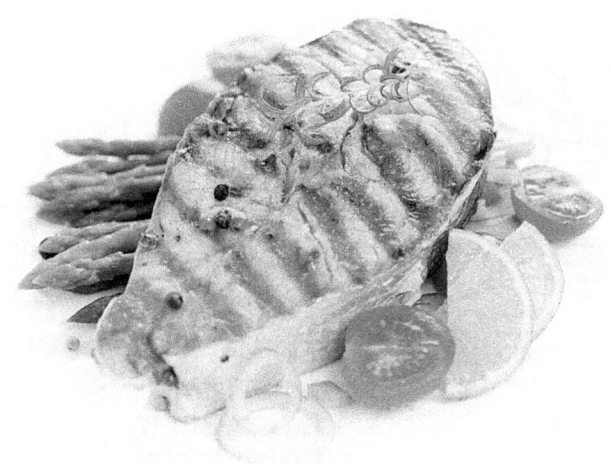

THE HARD STUFF

When we talk about spirits, we are talking about liquor. The word liquor is technically defined as "an alcoholic beverage made by distillation rather than by fermentation." As different as all the advertisers would have you believe their brand is, our body can't readily distinguish between single barrel and triple distillation, once the alcohol has passed your tongue, and hit the bloodstream.

If you've ever stepped into one of those liquor warehouse stores on your way to a party, you know how hopeless it can seem to even begin to talk about what sets all the different types and brands of liquor apart, but you've got to start some-where. And that "somewhere" for this discussion is: ingredients!

There are a variety of ingredients used as the base for liquors. Vodka usually starts with potatoes; bour-bon comes from corn; brandy starts out as fruit; rum uses sugar cane; tequila is made from blue agave, (commonly thought of as cactus—it is not); and so on and so on. Other spirits get their flavor from

TIPsy

Remember what we said about "well" drinks?
Well, you get what you pay for.

ingredients added after the fermentation of water, grain, and yeast. In the case of gin, for example, juniper berries give it that unique and pungent taste.

Distillation involves heating the mash produced by fermentation to a specific temperature, and then allowing it to condense back into liquid. After the first distillation has removed some of the impurities, the methanol (bad alcohol) is discarded, and everything is distilled again at a higher temperature, where the desired ethanol (good alcohol) is evaporated and condensed. Some spirits are distilled again and again to remove as many impurities as possible.

These impurities are called *congeners*, and they can vary in relative volume and content according to the type of liquor. Your body has to perform different chemical processes to filter out each one of these kinds of congeners, and that is one primary reason why it is not a great idea to mix liquors when you drink. The darker the alcohol, the more congeners it contains. And remember the top two contributing factors to a hangover are sugar and congeners.

Lighter colored spirits, such as vodka, gin, and some rums and tequilas, are not barrel-aged. They are stored in metal tanks, or simply bottled right after distillation.

A Little Sip of Each

*Nutritional Note: the vast majority of liquor varies between 96 and 103 calories per 1.5oz serving (a typical shot)

The Healthy Lush

Whiskey: Whiskey must be aged for a minimum of two years in new, white oak barrels that have been charred. Scotch and Bourbon's are similarly treated, and easily fall under this general definition. Some Doctor's colleagues at the EuroMedLab Scotland found that whiskey contains more ellagic acid than other types of alcohol, providing even more cancer cell-fighting antioxidants.

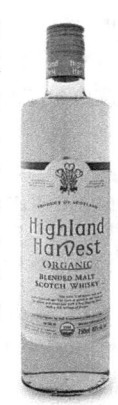

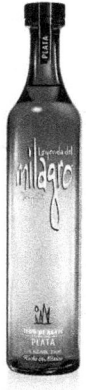

Tequila: Tequila is a regional name for a spirit called mescal, which is made only from blue agave plants. According to Mexican law, distilled tequila must be aged at least 8-10 years in oak barrels. In fact, Mexican law is very strict when it comes to the making of tequila. The process is not to be taken lightly. Tequila has been known to burn fat reserves which may be why it can make some people's clothes fall off!

TIPsy

Always choose tequilla made from 100% pure agave.
A good test is rub it on your hands it should turn oily not sticky...

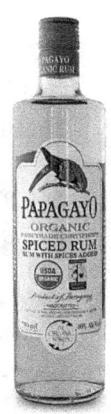

Rum: Rum is made through a fermentation process from cane sugar. The clear rums are either not aged at all, or aged slightly in metal tanks. Darker rums are aged longer, in wooden barrels. There is nothing more tasty than a Pina Colada made with premium dark rum! According to some research it's been found that moderate rum drinkers had a 38% lower risk of kidney cancer than those who didn't drink at all.

Gin: Gin: Like rum, gin makers have their own secret flavor recipes. Fancy ingredients include juniper berries, orange peel, cardamom, cassia bark, coriander, and angelica root. Besides being a lighter alcohol that is less likely to give you a hangover.

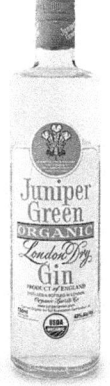

Premium Gin may have some other health benefits. Not only does it have less calories than some other liquors it is said to be the best natural remedy for arthritis. You may have heard of the old time remedy our parents used; gin soaked raisins. Well it is actually true!

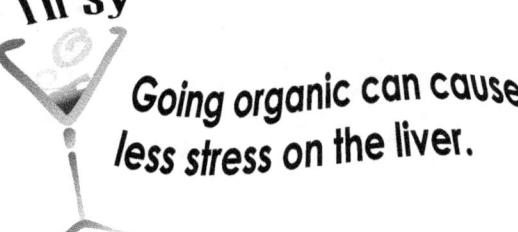

TIPsy

Going organic can cause less stress on the liver.

The Healthy Lush

Vodka: Modern vodka is perhaps the purest form of popular alcohol. The plain versions of vodka are distilled multiple times, and then filtered through charcoal, which removes almost all flavor and aroma. This is why vodka is such a popular base for mixed drinks, as it does not significantly affect the flavor. When it comes to organic alcohol, vodka is the most prevalent spirit that we could find that can be certified organic. Some may think the biggest health benefit of Vodka is that it can't be detected on their breath on their breath when they get home to their spouse!

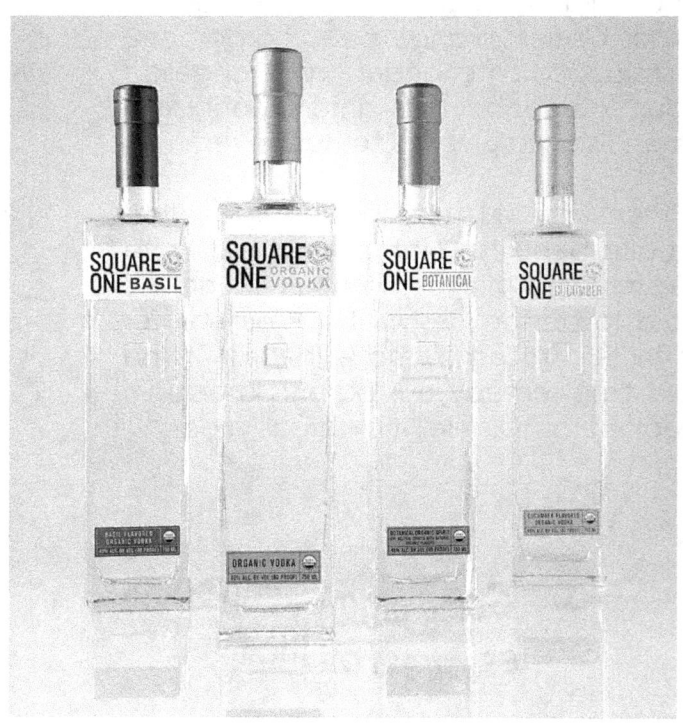

Mixers

Some mixers contain alcohol themselves, but most do not. As a general rule, we don't ever drink anything that's been premixed and sold in one big colorful bottle. All this means is they've added a little bit of liquor, tons of sugar, and some food coloring. You are much better off making the drinks yourself and controlling the ingredients. Besides being more health conscious, mixing and inventing your own tasty beverage is WAY more fun!

Vermouth is a popular mixer in martinis, which used to be made with gin as the base, but which are now made with all kinds of base liquors. The recipe is some big damn secret, but it usually contains things like marjoram, chamomile, cardamom, and cinnamon. Vermouth contains about sixteen percent alcohol, so do be aware it's adding to the alcoholic content of your drink, and drink wisely.

Bitters is another common alcoholic mixer. You wouldn't know it by the name, but Bitters contains sugar. One ounce has a whopping 135 calories and 4 grams of sugar. But the good news is that Bitters is not designed to be ingested by itself, only added in small amounts for flavor.

Cola might be the next most popular mixer. The problem here is the sugar and added calories. Did you know a Jack and Coke contains 173 calories and 10 grams of sugar? Imagine you drink three of these in one sitting. Your blood sugar will go through the roof, giving you a nasty headache, and making you super hungry. Ask the bartender if there is a diet soda available as a mixer instead. This is the lesser of two evils, but it is still better than regular cola.

Triple Sec (meaning "triple distilled") is a strong, sweet, colorless orange-flavored liqueur used as an ingredient in many mixed cocktails. It is made from the dried peel of oranges found on Curacao, an island in the Caribbean. Curacao, Grand Marnier, and Cointreau are other popular brands. One ounce of Triple Sec contains 105 calories and 11 grams of sugar! Some good substitutes are fresh squeezed orange juice, club soda, or a splash of Diet Sprite.

Sweet and sour mix is a blend of lemon juice and syrup. One ounce contains 30 calories and 8 grams of sugar. Most drink recipes that call for sweet and sour mix include more than a single ounce so, if you are counting calories, you can double those numbers...at least! A good substitute is a mixture of fresh squeezed lemon and lime juice, artificial sweetener, and then a dash of the real thing to get the right flavor. FYI, Baja Bob's makes a decent sugar-free sweet and sour mix.

Simple syrup is made of one-part water and one-part sugar. Simple syrup is commonly used in mixed cocktails such as lemon drops, mojitos, and other popular drinks one might find on a restaurant cocktail menu. An average serving of simple syrup contains 90 calories and up to 23 grams of sugar PER DRINK!

Many drink recipes call for simple syrup. Here is a version which works in those drink recipes, but is diabetic (and waistline) friendly. Use this wherever a recipe calls for simple syrup.

<u>Sugar-Free Simple Syrup Recipe</u>
1 cup sucralose sweetener (or even better Stevia. A natural herb sweetner)
1 cup boiling water
Dissolve sugar substitute in boiling water, and allow liquid to cool. Strain through a coffee filter to remove sediment.

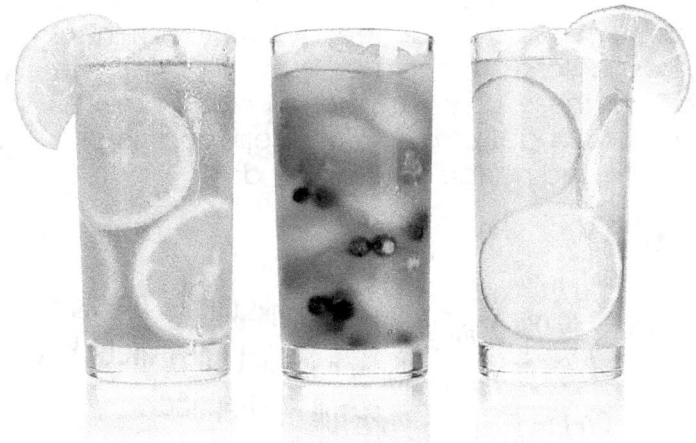

Stevia or other substitutes are great because they don't cause a spike in blood sugar, which can contribute to hangovers and binging. However, they can be a lot sweeter than sugar, and can disguise the taste of alcohol. Make and taste your simple syrup first, before adding alcohol.

Energy drinks These are the ones that promise to give its drinkers wings. These drinks claim to stimulate the mind and body, plus provide a boost of energy, but they can have adverse effects when mixed with alcohol. Instead of taking flight, you may be grounded if you have too many of these in one sitting. Energy drinks have stimulants in them that work in direct opposition to the depressive effect of alcohol. This nervous system conflict can contribute to a misperception of your level of impairment.

One 8-ounce can of Red Bull has 106 calories, 26 grams of sugar, and 77 milligrams of caffeine (WOW!). Our advice, if you feel compelled to use an energy drink as your mixer of choice, is to at least switch to a sugar-free version, to eliminate the excess calories and sugar. Also, only drink one. Do not use these as your mixer all night, or else your body won't get proper REM sleep, and you'll have a really bad hangover the next day.

TIPsy

In our opinion, energy drinks are the absolute WORST mixer, diet or non-diet. They wreak havoc on the liver, and are full of chemicals.

Rose's Lime Juice is a brand of sweetened, concentrated lime juice. It is commonly used in mixed cocktails such as kamikazes and cosmopolitans. It's good at disguising the taste of alcohol and sugar in a drink. One ounce contains 8 calories, 3 grams of carbohydrates and a half gram of sugar. A good substitute is juice from a fresh squeezed lime, and a dash of a sugar substitute, if needed.

Grenadine is a sugar syrup made from red currants and pomegranates. It is a useful ingredient for many cocktails, acting as both a coloring agent and a sweetener. One ounce contains 75 calories and 19 grams of sugar! A good substitute is fresh pomegranate juice, a splash of diet soda, and red food coloring if you want to add color.

Juice is a commonly mistaken for a healthy mixer. Fruit juice is generally full of sugar, especially the kind of juice you'll typically find at a bar. A good general rule is to avoid it completely, or use only a splash of it as a sweetener. An 8-ounce glass of regular orange juice contains an average of 115 calories, 30 grams of carbs, and 22 grams of sugar! Fresh squeezed juice is always a better choice, because it doesn't have any added sugar or corn syrup.

The good news about juice is citrus fruits contain high levels of vitamin C and zinc, which are both proven to help in avoiding a hangover.

Carbonated water, which includes soda water, club soda, seltzer, and sparkling water, are all good choices for mixers. Make sure they have no added sugar or chemicals. But remember; alcohol, when mixed with carbonated beverages, is absorbed more quickly than when mixed with non-carbonated beverages.

Food Pairings

Food pairings are the same with most alcohol: the same things we know are good for us when we are NOT drinking are good for us when we ARE drinking. The problem is, we forget what those things are when we are out at happy hour, so we will remind you once again:

BEST

1. Shellfish: lobster, crab, shrimp, clams, mussels

2. Fish: swordfish, salmon, halibut

3. Chicken: high in protein and B vitamins

4. Turkey: high in protein, low in fat, and contains niacin, selenium, and B vitamins

5. Sushi: contains amino acids, omega-3

6. Green vegetables: fiber (duh!)

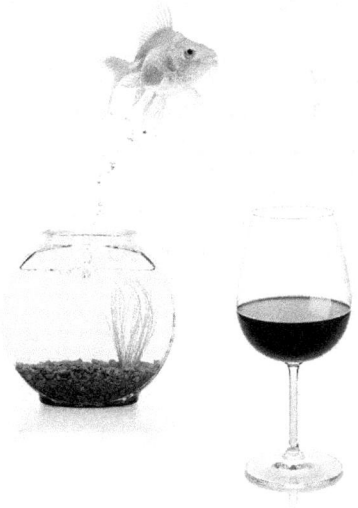

GOOD

1. Steak: protein, but higher in fat, and harder for your body to digest

2. Pasta: high in amino acids, and helps put nutrients back in your body, and quickly fills your stomach to help absorb the alcohol

3. Cheese: high in protein and calcium, but also high in fat

4. Bread: as with pasta, it will fill your stomach, and help slow the absorption process, but pick a whole-grain bread, not white, and add a small amount of butter for a fat source

5. Fruit: contains antioxidants, but be careful not to eat too much, because fruit is high in sugar, and a bad combination with already sugary drinks

6. Yogurt: high in protein, low in fat, but choose a light brand, with no added corn syrup, and go organic if possible

7. Pizza: try to only have one slice, but the amino acids, protein and fat from the cheese are better than eating nothing

TIPsy

Good, unsaturated fat, rather than high-sugar carbs, are much better for you while drinking. So put some butter on that bread!

The Healthy Lush

Nuts: protein, contain a lot of necessary vitamins and minerals, and they're easy to eat, but be careful because they're high in fat

WORST

1. Chips: saturated fat, digested quickly, and contain no nutrients

2. Candy: too much sugar, and no need to add extra calories. (You already chose to do that by drinking alcohol.)

3. Potatoes: no nutritional value in mashed potatoes and absorbed quickly

4. Ice cream: stay away from anything too high in sugar, or limit the number of mouthfuls you slurp up.

5. White Bread: has minimal nutritional value and will create a spike in blood sugar, which will contribute to the dreaded hangover.

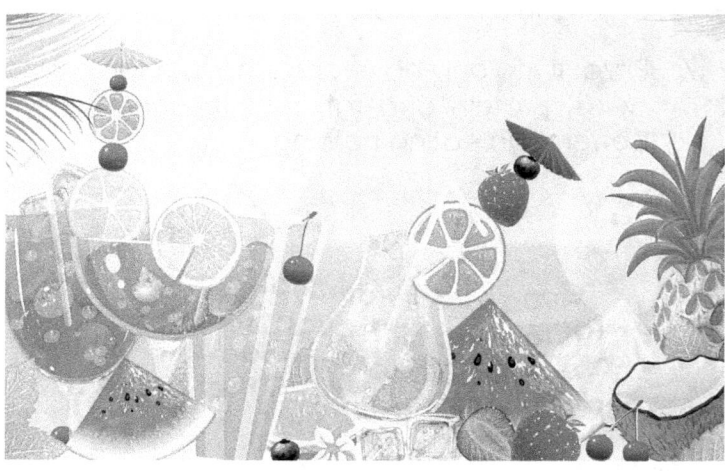

Froo-Froo Drinks

These are the drinks that come with umbrellas!

You can order them even when you're not on the beach, ya know. It's adorable.

And that's all we've got to say about that...

The Short and Sweet of It

The most important thing to note about all of the above is that they contain elevated levels of sugar. Have we mentioned sugar yet? Added sugar means carbs, calories, trips to the dentist, and worst of all, alterations by your tailor. That is not to mention the potential health risks associated with consuming too much refined sugar.

One of the risks worth a special mention is a condition called: hypoglycemia. Functional hypoglycemia is caused by a diet high in refined carbohydrates. Eating or drinking sugar-laden stuff causes your blood sugar levels to rise rapidly, which signals and stimulates the pancreas to secrete an excess of insulin. This excess insulin works to remove too much sugar from the blood, which can create an abnormally low blood-sugar level.

Here are some guidelines to help avoid it:

1. Do not drink more than two drinks of alcohol in a twenty-four hour period. As we said at the beginning, one drink is a 12-ounce beer, a 5-ounce glass of wine or a 1.5-ounce shot of liquor.

The Healthy Lush

2. Drink alcohol only with food.

3. Drink slowly.

4. Avoid sugary mixed drinks, sweet wines, and cordials.

5. Mix liquor with water, or diet soft drinks.

Sounds like good advice in general. In general, good advice usually equates to not much fun—but it beats the heck out of giving yourself daily insulin injections, or worse. Remember this the next time you are pounding down those hard lemonades!

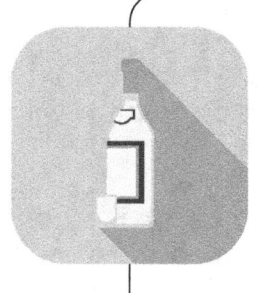

FUN FACT

The calorie content of a standard drink of beer, dinner wine, or distilled spirits (either straight or in a mixed drink) is equivalent. So if all you mean by "lightweight" is that your drink comes with an umbrella...give it up, sister. Nothing light about it!

In the (*ahem*) spirit of cutting down on your sugar intake, while still enjoying the tastes associated with various liqueurs, we'd like to offer some ideas for ingredient substitutes. You may need to experiment with the tastes, of course, but many of these have far fewer grams of sugar than the liqueurs they replace.

Substitute Suggestions:

- **Amaretto:** Amaretto is said to taste like almonds, but, interestingly, contains none. Nevertheless, the perfect substitution for amaretto is almond extract. As almond extract has a much stronger flavor, only use about a quarter of the amount of amaretto called for.

- **Bourbon:** A teaspoon or two of nonalcoholic vanilla extract

- **Brandy:** Try fruit juices, water, cherry syrup (from canned cherries), white grape juice, or apple juice

- **Champagne:** Sparkling fruit juices such as apple, grape, or cranberry. Also, try ginger ale

- **Coffee Liqueur:** Espresso, coffee syrup, nonalcoholic coffee extract

- **Cognac:** Pear, peach, or apricot juice

- **Crème de menthe:** Spearmint extract or spearmint oil, diluted

- **Ouzo:** Anise Italian soda syrup (sugar free, of course)

- **Peach Brandy:** Syrup from canned peaches; try to find sugar-free or lite versions

- **Peppermint Schnapps:** Mint leaves, or nonalcoholic peppermint extract

- **Port wine:** Concord grape juice, orange, or apple juice

The Healthy Lush

- **Red wine:** Cranberry juice, grape juice, tomato juice, beef or vegetable broth

- **Rum:** Vanilla extract, or nonalcoholic rum; also, try pineapple or apple juice

- **Sherry:** Apple, pineapple, and orange juice, or peach syrup

- **Good sense:** There is no substitute for common sense when it comes to drinking healthily. But you've already got plenty of it if you're reading the end of this chapter. Apply your good sense in liberal portions, and that will be the recipe for your good health. Bottoms up!

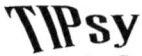

TIPsy

When it comes to alcohol women and men are definitely not equal. Women tend to get drunk more quickly, and stay drunk longer than men.

IN AN ALCOHOLIC NUTSHELL

Alcohol Content

Think about the alcohol content of the liquor you're using. The general rule when it comes to alcohol proof is that the higher the proof, the greater the alcohol content, and the greater the calorie-count.

Eighty-proof alcohol is the most widely available, and it is made up of forty percent alcohol, and 100-proof alcohol is fifty percent alcohol. When you make your own low-calorie alcoholic drinks, it's important to take note of the proof, so you know how many calories you're getting per ounce of liquor.

Beer

If you enjoy beer, then your best bet for a low-calorie alcoholic drink is light beer. Light beer can reduce your calorie count by up to half in some cases. Most light beer has approximately four percent alcohol, while regular beer has an alcohol content of five percent or more. Some pale ales and light lagers however, have an alcohol content as low as three and a half percent; these are the best low-calorie alcoholic drinks because a 12-ounce bottle has just 95 calories.

Some beer manufacturers have gone even further, to offer you the lowest-calorie alcoholic drinks with brands like Miller 64, which has just 64 calories, and Budweiser Select, which has 55 calories.

Wine/Champagne

The key to enjoying low-calorie alcoholic drinks like wine is portion size. Wine doesn't have a lot of calories, but the calories can truly add up when the amounts consumed aren't monitored.

Our favorite bar or restaurant can serve glasses as large as eight fluid ounces, which means 188 calories in a glass.

Spirits

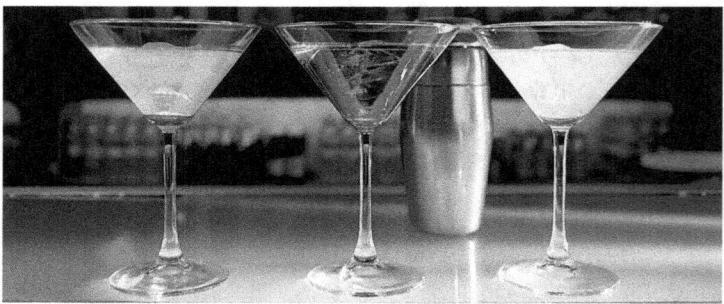

Drinking spirits, also known as hard liquor, is your best option for creating low-calorie alcoholic drinks. Whether you enjoy spirits on the rocks, or blended with a mixer, you can enjoy a low-calorie alcoholic drink with just 103 calories per serving.

Most people believe that hard alcohol is the most troublesome for weight loss, but nothing could be further from the truth. Let's take gin for example, which has just 96 calories per serving. If you enjoy gin on the rocks, or with a splash of lime, you can enjoy one of the lowest-calorie alcoholic drinks, with just 96 calories.

Other types of alcohol, like vodka, tequila, and rum, range in calorie count from 97 to 103 calories per 1.5 ounce serving. To take these spirits, and create low-calorie alcoholic drinks requires you to make smarter choices about what you mix with it.

Low Calorie Mixers

Gin and (diet) tonic is one of the lowest-calorie alcoholic drinks you can have, with just 96 calories!

Creating low-calorie alcoholic drinks often comes down to what goes in the glass with the alcohol.

Soda: If you're a rum and coke, or gin and tonic drinker, swap out the high-calorie soda for diet soda. Diet cola and diet tonic water have zero calories, so you can enjoy a gin and tonic that has just 96 calories.

Juice: Choose fresh-squeezed juice over sugary, high-calorie juices. To make a low-calorie screwdriver, squeeze the juice from one orange rather than using orange juice with added sugar. Simply Orange and Odwalla are good alternatives.

Avoid alcoholic drinks that have more than one or two types of alcohol in them, because the calorie count (and alcohol content) will be too high. Keep liqueurs and syrups to a minimum as well, if you want a low-calorie alcoholic drink.

The Healthy Lush

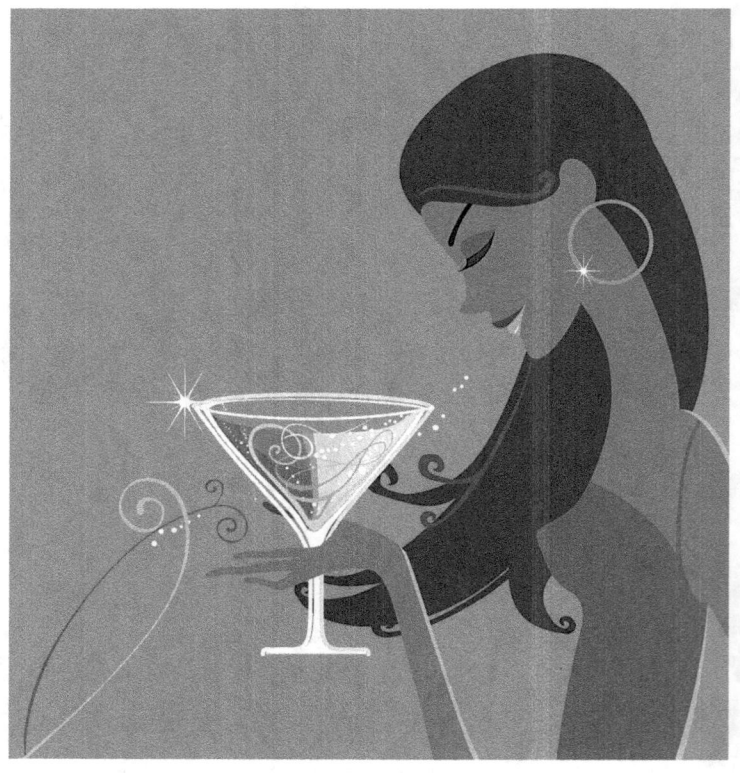

HEALTHY LUSH FAVORITES

In our travels, we've tried to find nice adult beverages that have some healthy ingredients. It's been tough doing all this field research.. but hey, someone's got to do it! We took the bullet for you. Here's what we've learned:

Mojito (This version is our own invention.)

White rum
Sparkling water
Agave nectar
Mint
Freshly squeezed lime juice

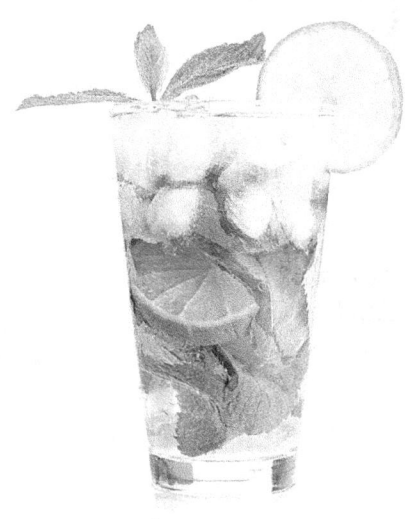

The Healthy Lush

Cucumber Cooler
(from the VeeV website, http://veevlife.com/)

VeeV açai spirit
Three sliced cucumbers, muddled
Soda water

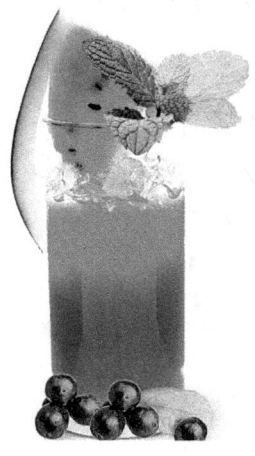

Acai Watermelon Cooler
(we can't remember)

VeeV açai spirit
Fresh watermelon juice
Muddled mint
Club soda
Blueberries

LIV IT UP (LIV at the Fontainebleau in Miami)

1.5 ounces premium vodka
½ ounce peach schnapps
2 ounces sugar-free Redbull
2 ounces soda
Squeeze of lemon

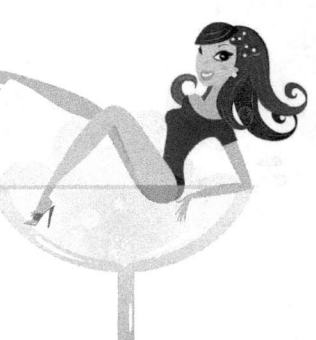

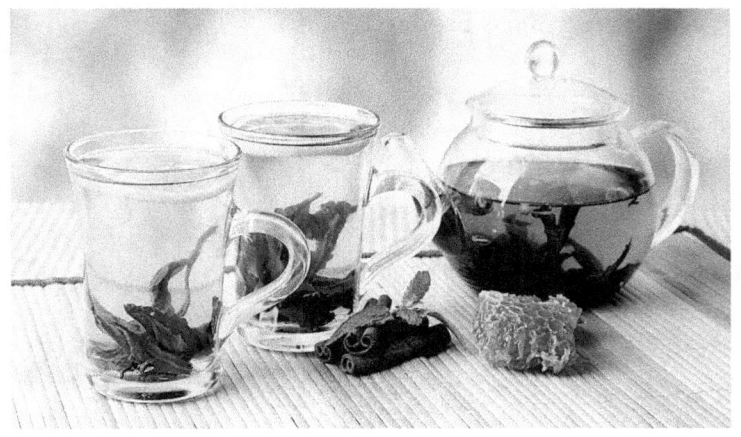

Green Tea Hot Toddy
(Fran Drescher, from *Rachel Ray* magazine)

1 tablespoon honey
¾ cup hot brewed green tea
¼ cup whiskey
Lemon for garnish, and to taste

The Ruby (*Spirit* magazine)

¾ pound red beets, peeled and liquefied
½ liter vodka
1 part sugar (We recommend using a
sugar substitute, in moderation.)
1 part water
¼ ounce lemon juice
¼ ounce lime juice

Blueberry Citrus Breeze*

10 blueberries
¾ ounce liquid Stevia
(vanilla flavored
works good too)
1 1/2 ounces Juniper
Green Organic Gin
3/4 ounce fresh
squeezed lemon juice
Splash of champagne

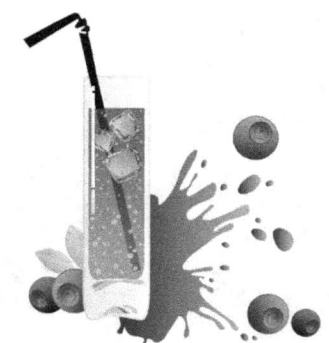

In a shaker, muddle together blueberries and stevia. Add the gin and lemon juice, Strain contents of shaker into a martini glass and then top with champagne.*

The Wolper

Fill short glass completely with ice cubes (don't skimp on the ice it actually loosens the aromatic molecules and heightens rather than dilutes the flavor)

Pour glass 2/3rds full of Square
One Organic Vodka
Squeeze ½ lime and ¼ lemon in glass
Add splash of roses lime juice (to taste)

Or the classic....

Pickle-Back
(Burning Man Cosmic Recess)
Large shot of Irish whiskey
Pickle juice (any brand will do)

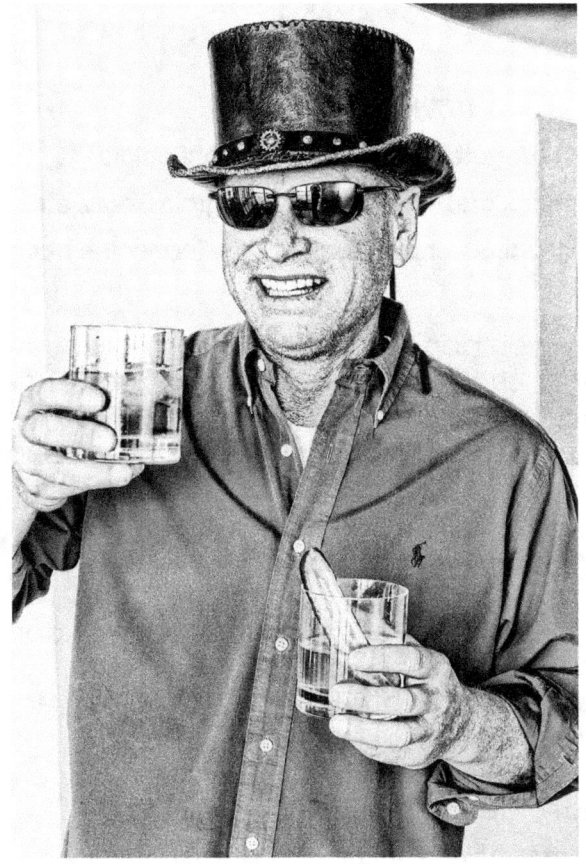

Robby Stowe, *Cover Artist*

A VERY SHORT CHAPTER

Failing To Plan is Not Planning...oops!

Bottoms Up Food Pyramid
5% Alcohol

10% Fat

10% Fruit: berries, etc.

15% Vegetables: green and bright colors

20% Complex carbohydrates: whole grains, oats, etc.

40% Protein: animal or plant based... the leaner the better

We know you don't wake up every morning and think, "What should I have with me, in case I get drunk tonight?" Neither do we. Yet when we know there is an occasion or event planned, and we know we'll be drinking, it's easier to plan for a healthier approach. For example, we make sure we take our supplements. (Read the earlier chapters...)

But there is always that unexpected party, happy hour, or any other version of an excuse to drink with friends, and then what? First, decide if it is really worth it. Ask yourself;

1. Is that cute guy/gal going to be there?

2. Will they be serving your favorite peanut M&Ms?

3. Will attending this event mean anything to your career?

4. Can you sneak out undetected if it's awful?

5. Paper or plastic?

If you answered yes to any two of those then yes, you have to go!

First of all...EAT! Even a small amount will save you a big amount of potential embarrassment and pain the next day. Eat something small, but nutrient dense so the alcohol doesn't go immediately to your head (or your liver) and make you pig out on high-calorie bar food.

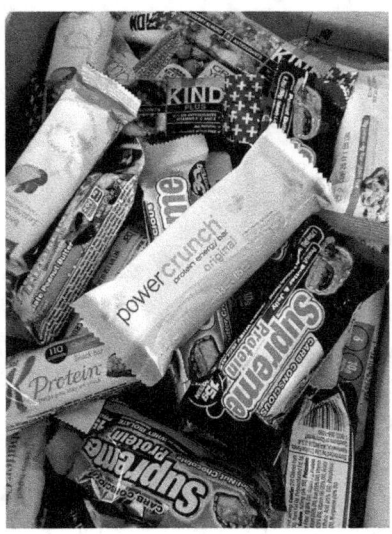

Here are some quick suggestions:

• A slice of turkey wrapped in lettuce leaves

• A mini-bag of popcorn and an orange

• Veggie sticks with hummus and tofu

The Healthy Lush

- Handful of almonds or mixed nuts

- Yogurt sprinkled with flaxseed

- Fiber or protein bar

- String cheese

- Small bowl of high-fiber cereal

- A cup of lentil soup...you can keep instant soups in your office

- A half-cup cottage cheese

- Whole-wheat, high-fiber crackers with cheese or peanut butter

- Beef or turkey jerky

Some of these are easy to keep in your purse or office drawer, just in case you get that text inviting you out, at which point you realize you haven't eaten all day.

If you have time you can make Holistic Gourmet Brain Balls! They are amazing and can keep you healthy all day any time.

Brain Balls
1 cup almond butter...peanut butter or nut butter of your choice
1 cup chopped soaked organic walnuts
1 cup chopped soaked organic almonds

1 cup chopped soaked organic pumpkin seeds
½ cup chia seeds ground (optional)
½ cup ground flax seeds
1 cup hemp seeds
1 cup ground gogi berries (optional)
1 tbs maca root (optional)
2 tbs coconut oil (softened)
2 tbs of raw honey
2 tsp almond extract or vanilla
1 tsp sea salt
1 cup shredded coconut

Use soaked nuts if possible (dry well after soaking) or regular organic nuts and seeds...

Chop nuts and seeds separately in a small cuisinart... Grind gogi berries and chia seeds (I use a coffee grinder for these)

Mix all ingredients together... Roll into golf sized balls and roll in coconut

Store in fridge...will last about about 2 weeks... enjoy...yum!!!

Makes about 30 balls*

*The Holistic Gourmet *High Vibe Recovery

www.patireiss.com

TIPsy

If you drink regularly, we recommend a daily detox: drink a cup of hot water with the juice of half a lemon each morning

THE HANGOVER

or I Swear, I'll Never Do That Again!

Even armed with this simple wisdom and a plan to practice moderation, it is easy to fall victim to the priority re-engineering demon that often appears after that third Long Island Iced Tea. There are ways to minimize the post-party effects caused by having too much of a good thing; otherwise technically known as: "*Veisalgia*". The roots of this word come from the Norwegian word for "uneasiness following debauchery" (*kevis*) and the Greek word for "pain" (*algia*). You might unaffectionately recognize it as ... **the hangover.**

Here is one scenario where the saying, "The greater the journey, the greater the reward," is NOT going to be applicable. There is no physical reward for a night of heavy debauchery. Well at least not one that alcohol is going to give you.

There is NOTHING worse than the feeling of an awful hangover. We have ALL been here, done this...and never want to look back. The older you get, the worse the hangovers get. In your twenties, you could throw back eighteen beers, two bottles of water, drink the frat boy next to you under the table with tequila shots, and still wake up the next day with only an almost undetectable headache. Not so much as you get older. Eventually a subtle glass of wine will make you feel like you're knocking on death's door. So, for all of you hangover-prone drinkers...here's some advice to live by.

AVOID THE HANGOVER in the first place by following the practices we've just taught you. We feel hung over not from the alcohol itself, but from the process of it leaving our bodies...much like the withdrawal experienced by a recovering drug addict, or sugar addict—or pretty much anything else we choose to overindulge in.

Here are a few quick hints for avoiding hangovers:

1. Drink no more than three liquor based drinks in one sitting.

2. Sip each drink slowly to allow your body time to filter out the impurities gradually.

3. Stick with one kind of liquor for the duration of the night.

4. Drink lots of water. Either mix it in, or have a glass of water between drinks.

5. Take glutamine supplements after you drink, to help you sleep.

6. Organic liquor is better. Check the label, or ask if it's available.

7. Take a multi-vitamin.

Our favorite:

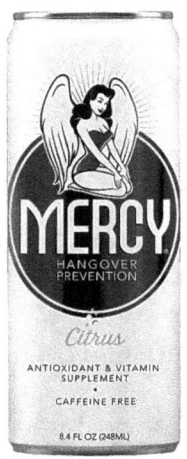

And if you haven't listened to us at all...

TIPsy

Mercy contains L-Cysteine, an amino acid that helps release alcohol-resolving enzymes in the liver and dissolve the acetaldehyde that is the primary cause of a hangover.

HOW TO CURE A HANGOVER

There are a lot of products on the market that claim to "cure" the common hangover. First, let's check out some (sometimes true and accurate) old wives' tales.

Hair of the dog

Doesn't it make sense that if too much alcohol made you feel bad, then more alcohol will not make you feel better? The only thing drinking again will do is delay the inevitable. Just put your tail between your legs and whimper through it. However, hangover effects begin to manifest 11+ hours after your last cocktail. It's the effect of the body struggling to eliminate the various impurities and trying to get back to normal after the alcohol's left the body. If you are truly struggling and need to delay the inevitable do it gently. Try the **Hangover Hydrator** (from Zest Bar SLC, UT); Coconut Water with Organic chocolate vodka. It's yummy and might help you get through the day.

Burnt Toast

There is a professed theory is that the carbon in burnt toast works like activated charcoal to help filter the alcohol out of your system. While activated charcoal is indeed used to filter some poisons, it is not used to treat alcohol poisoning. Moreover, carbon from burnt toast is not the same thing as activated charcoal. Try taking a tablespoon of activated charcoal instead. Burnt toast might be able to justify your craving a pre-dawn trip to the diner, but it won't help you with a hangover. Speaking of diners...

The Healthy Lush

Fried or Fatty Foods

"Eat some fried chicken and pie!" Uncle Earl always recommended for a hangover. Meanwhile, Uncle Earl is four hundred pounds, and has a cardiologist on speed dial. No thanks!

Eating fried or fatty foods <u>before</u> you drink might actually be more beneficial. Not only do they minimize the effects of alcohol by slowing down absorption, but also fatty and greasy foods in particular will coat the stomach lining for a bit longer than other, healthier foods. Eating bad food after you drink will only irritate your stomach more.

Not to "bring up" your meal but…

Puking (voluntary or otherwise)

This seems like the worst option, but it's actually one of the best. The sooner you get the alcohol out of your system the better! Just remember that by the time your stomach is irritated enough to make you want to vomit, the alcohol has most likely already been absorbed into your bloodstream. Throw up,

TIPsy

If you stop drinking two or three hours before you go to sleep, you won't wake up with a huge hangover.
We (almost) guarantee it!

hydrate yourself, and eat something nutritious as soon as you are able to keep down food again. Oh, and be sure to flush...twice!

Coffee

Nobody likes a wide-awake drunk. Besides, coffee is a diuretic. Even though it's made with water, coffee actually dehydrates you. It won't hurt you to drink some coffee, but it's definitely not going to help hydrate you.

Brushing Your Teeth

We also heard that brushing your teeth before you go to bed cures a hangover as well. LOL, seriously? This sounds like some deviant plot by a mom with alcoholic children to manipulate them into cleanliness. We can't say that this is going to work for sure but we CAN for sure say that NOT brushing your teeth before you go to bed is just gross and unhygienic. And there's a possibility that it could ruin your social life!

Cold Shower

Ah, the old cold shower trick is yet another cure! There's no question that a cold shower will rehydrate you. Your skin will drink in the water and replace a little bit of the moisture lost from drinking. Most of our water loss happens through urination, but some of it is lost through the skin as sweat. Don't forget, the skin is an organ too. It needs proper hydration just as much as your internal organs. If possible, soak the skin with a nice shower, bath or swim before bedtime. Be sure to wear your floaties. Oh, and use the buddy system.

Raw Eggs

This is just gross, but we've heard that it works... You can try it and let us know! We prefer the 2am Denny's run. Eggs actually can help. They contain large amounts of cysteine, the substance that breaks down the hangover-causing toxin acetaldehyde in the liver's easily depleted glutathione.

OTC Products

We'll refrain from discussing any specific over-the-counter products. What we will say is if you're taking a capsule of some kind, and drinking it down with a big glass of water, then you're doing yourself a world of good...with the water. If the product you're taking also happens to include B vitamins, glutamine, electrolytes, or anything else you depleted by drinking, all the better.

However...

We have had some personal success with taking ibuprofen.

Ibuprofen works by blocking the production of prostaglandins, a type of cyclic fatty acid that cause pain and swelling (inflammation). They are released in the brain and can cause headaches. Unfortunately, these prostaglandins are also released when excess alcohol is consumed.

We have found that taking 400 milligrams just before bed time can help prevent those dreaded head and body aches we feel the morning after a night of fun. It is not harmful to take another 400 mg in the morning if the symptoms are still present. Please contact your doctor before taking any over the counter medication and always follow the directions on the bottle... too bad liquor bottles don't give us dosage directions!

Hangover Cure Recipes

The Healthy Lush Cure

1 banana
1 cup fresh squeezed orange juice
6 strawberries
1 cup organic, unsweetened soy milk
Dash nutmeg
1 packet Emergen-C
3 egg whites
Ice
Blend all ingredients, and enjoy!

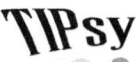

TIPsy

"One of the quickest ways to cure a hangover is to make a banana milkshake." From a newspaper in Mysore, India, the center for yoga and holistic healing
- also, a dry country...hmm.

The Healthy Lush

Easy Cure Bloody Mary

5 oz tomato juice
3 oz light beer
Salt and pepper
Lots of lime juice
Dash of Tabasco sauce
Mix, and serve over ice

Sauerkraut Hangover Soup

1 small onion, chopped
1 teaspoon paprika
2 cups water
3 cups chicken or vegetable stock
1 green pepper, shredded
1 tomato, chopped
16 ounces sauerkraut
1 tablespoon flour
1 cup sour cream
½ pound spicy smoked sausage (can substitute turkey bacon, or tofu)

Throw all ingredients into slow cooker, and cook on low for six hours. If possible, let it cook overnight, so it's ready for the morning!

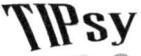

TIPsy

The first miracle hangover cure we found...
Remember all those B vitamins?
One large shot of this in the morning,
followed by some kombucha tea,
canhelp get you through the day!

Zinc Slaw
(Nutritional Self Defense by Sheridan Goulart)

10 carrots, grated
½ c sunflower seeds
½ c alfalfa sprouts
¼ c wheat germ
½ c each red and green cabbage

Quinoa Super~Food Salad
(The Holistic Gourmet – Pati Reiss)

3 cups of cooked quinoa (1c quinoa 2 c water)
1 cup fresh blueberries
1 cup gogi berries
1 c sunflower seeds
1 ½ cups of chopped kale lacinato my favorite
1 cup edaname beans
1 acai smoothie packet or ¾ cup of acai juice
2-4 limes
1-2 oranges

Cook quinoa...chop kale then either blanch it in hot salted water for about 3 minutes then drain or sauté in olive oil with a splash of apple juice...add to quinoa in a large mixing bowl...add blueberries, sunflowers, gogi berries and edaname beans...mix the acai smoothie pack or juice in blender with fresh lime and orange juice...slowly add to salad... mix together and eat...Enjoy!!!

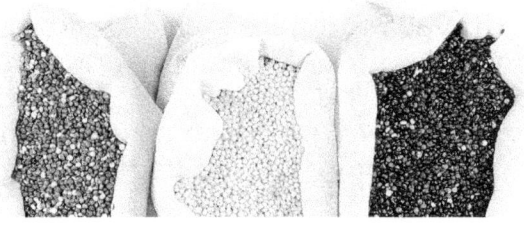

Our Number One Hangover Cure

Take a huge shot of E3
Immediately and quickly drink one kombucha tea.
Lie down for thirty minutes. You'll feel the difference!
(be careful with this one if you have a sulphite allergy)

⊚ E3Live®

Komubucha is well known for its detoxifying and digestive enzymes and can be extremely helpful curing that hangover nausea.

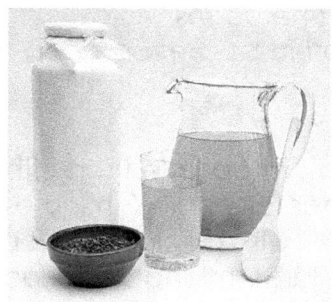

The best time to address a hangover is to take steps to avoid one before you start drinking. The next best time is while you are drinking. The worst time, and also when most people think about it, is when you're done drinking, or the next day. Everyone seems to have his or her own cure for a hangover. Since the hangover is only a collection of symptoms, there really is no cure. All you can really do the next day is to try to treat each symptom.

The Rest Of The Story

In a perfect world, you didn't drink too much the night before. In a really good world, you planned ahead, followed our recommendations, and you're only experiencing mild suffering. In a pretty-darned-good world, you don't have to work, or function the next day. Unfortunately, in the real world, you probably have no choice but to get up, and get going.

While we strongly recommend resting your body, too much rest can be unhealthy. So take the opportunity to burn off all those unwanted calories from the night before by "exercising" your options. We tend to beat ourselves up when we've overindulged, but try not to wallow in it. Remember, the sooner you get back to your normal routine, the faster you'll get rid of those calories, and the better you'll feel about yourself mentally!

One pound on your frame is equivalent to 3500 calories. If you are consuming 3500 calories a day, and not burning that much, you are gaining weight. Relax though; most of us don't come close to consuming 3500 unburned calories a day under normal circumstances. On the other hand, those drinks you had last night (how many was it?!) didn't do you any favors.

Any physical activity is good. Start with rolling out of bed. Then use this handy guide to help you decide which exercise is right for you.

If what you drank last night was sweet, it was probably loaded with calories. It sucks, but anything that tastes good is probably bad for you. Now, you only have twenty-four hours to burn off those calories before they start being stored as fat. Here are some suggestions for post-alcoholic-indulgence exercise:

Swimming is good for re-hydrating, and the number one recommended exercise the morning after drinking. Swimming replenishes some of the water lost out of your skin and leaves you feeling refreshed. It's a great workout for your joints and anyone suffering from muscle pain. Swimming burns up to 280 calories in just one half-hour session. Swim for an hour, and you've burned over 500 calories, gotten a good dose of natural vitamin D, rehydrated your skin, and given your body the gift of a natural hangover cure!

Running: It's at the top for best calorie burn, and is an exercise you can do most anywhere. We call it the "no excuses exercise," because you should be able to get up and go running just about anywhere. Running burns anywhere from 600 to 1000 calories per hour depending on pace and weight and it tones every single muscle in your body. Problem is if you drank way too much, this might not be a good idea. It could end up making you feel worse than before.

Hiking: Hiking is a great way to get outside, get some sun and fresh air, and it's an activity you can make easy or strenuous depending on how you feel. Either way, it's a fun way to burn calories while being social at the same time.

Go to the gym: Most of us don't want to do it, ever,

let alone when we've had a few cocktails the night before. You know you will always feel better when you're done. Spend some time on a treadmill, bike, or elliptical machine. You'll sweat, burn calories, and wake yourself up. If you're feeling great, take a group class to motivate yourself.

Yoga: It might not be at the top of the list for calorie burning. It's hard to give an exact number because there are so many different types of yoga practices out there, but the stretching and twisting helps to wring out the organs, and rid your body of toxins.

Yoga can help move energy, and create increased circulation. The lymphatic system also gets activated, and that helps move some of the toxins out more quickly. It also helps calm the mind, and create a sense of peace.

Disclaimer: If you already have a hangover, be careful doing hot yoga! Remember your body is already dehydrated. Be sure to drink LOTS of water, and leave the room if you feel dizzy or too hot. Ann loves Ashtanga. The average woman can burn around 600 calories, and the average man around 900.

It's really up to you how you want to exercise, but you do need to do some kind of movement.

... And if you happen to be in Vegas and forgot everything we just said call **Hangover Heaven**. They will administer a vitamin drip that will make you good as new - www.hangoverheaven.com.

The Healthy Lush

Things to Avoid:

- Don't stay in bed all day (unless you're going to get some exercise there!)
- Avoid watching too much TV.
- No trips to fast food establishments.
- No grocery shopping! (You are probably craving unhealthy foods.)
- Watch out for excessive heat. Get some sun, but don't overdo it.
- No tanning beds

All things considered, the best way to deal with a hangover is to never have one. See, that's why you were supposed to start at the beginning of the book!

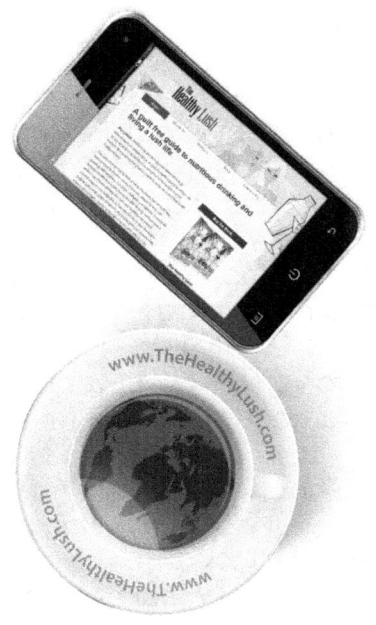

REVIEW

1. Alcohol: happiest accident ever!
2. Read this book from the beginning.
3. Don't drink on an empty stomach.
4. Drink water before, during, and after—all the time! Just drink water!
5. Too much refined sugar can make you feel like shhh...ugar
6. Take a bath.
7. Then take a shower.
8. Eat some eggs.
9. Moderate drinkers enjoy better health than nondrinkers.
10. Hangovers suck!
11. Exercise! Swim, run, hike, rob a bank...whatever gets you out of the house.
12. Try some of our recommended recipe
13. Don't drink and drive.
14. Congeners suck more than vampires.
15. Organic alcohol doesn't suck.
16. Seafood goes great with wine (especially when it's stuffed with asparagus, and topped with yogurt).
17. Vitamins and minerals are your good friends.
18. Water is your BFF.
19. Tut, tut, tut! There's alcohol in our pyramid!
20. Plan your spontaneity.

21. Curfews are for grown-up kids, too.

22. Have a designated carriage, or else your midnight pumpkin may be a three-hundred-pound cellmate.

23. Mexico takes tequila very seriously.

24. The number one cause of hangovers is dehydration.

25. Be HAPPY.

26. Buy this book for a friend!

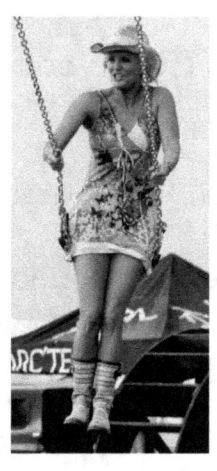

LAST CALL

Closing time! You don't have to go home but you can't stay here.

Okay, so by this point hope-fully you've had a little fun, paused for brief moments to stroll down memory lane as you're reading, thought about your favorite cocktail at your local bar, and learned a little along the way.

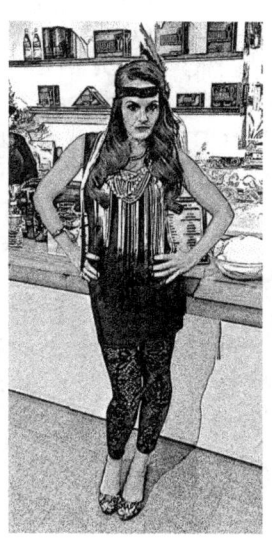

Now, none of us like the "al-ways gets wasted obnoxious drunk" hanging around but probably most of us have fond memories that still make us laugh till we cry when some-one (or somones...) got a little too drunk. We all have our stories... like the "walk of shame" only getting back to your room and find-ing the key to your room doesn't work! Or like our friend who got so intoxicated she parted the Asian Sea of tourists at Mandalay Bay because she had to be wheeled out of the casino in a wheel chair. But this one might just take the cake... it still keeps us laughing.

Here's one of our fun dinner stories

It was a Bachelorette party (you know who you are) and of course included an adult entertainment show for women in "Sin City"... champagne, limo ride etc. After a VERY steamy show and several

The Healthy Lush

cocktails we decided it was time to call it and night and head back to the ranch. Problem was, one of our friends (let's call her Anita Mann... she fortunately was NOT the Bachelorette) had made her way backstage, apparently to show her appreciation to one of the 'artists' in the show. Most likely 'Chip or Dale'... as she slipped past the curtain we slipped the address home in her pocket as she promised she would make it back on her own.

The rest of us jumped into the limo and took the scenic way home enjoying our limo and champagne. Imagine our surprise when arrived, opened the door and found one of the more attractive 'artists' we had just seen performing for us earlier... (lets call him Hugh Jorgan) rapidly wrapping a towel around his waste and "Anita" gasping with great surprise in the background.

Now any of you girls out there who have been to any of these male shows in Vegas and had a few too many cocktails can imagine what happened next. The girls began squealing and waving their hands like 11year olds at a New-Kids-on-the-Block concert as they lunged across the room at this poor, unsuspecting fellow.

Needless to say, our arrival and a potential encore performance caused him to rethink his well-laid plan. Or, perhaps, his plan to get well laid. We'll never know. "Hugh" high tailed it out of there before you could say premature ejaculation.

We laughed about it for weeks... actually years! In this case, it made for a good story and "Anita" was fine but then again, something bad could have happened to her (or maybe something good happened to her) you just never know.

We are glad we've all survived some of those crazy days. But mostly we just enjoy quiet conversations with friends and a great glass of wine, the cocktails on the beach, the occasional mornings we get to steal from our daily routine and pop open a bottle of champagne in bed with lox and bagel's, the bottles of wine we enjoy at our book clubs (ours is appropriately called 'Wine, Women and Words') and the toasts we get to share with the ones we love.

The most important thing to remember, above all things, as with any type of healthy living, is just to be mindful. Next time you're sitting at the local pub with girlfriends, and the hot bartender says, "What can I get ya?" THINK first. Tell them how to make your favorite drink the low-cal way, so that you can enjoy more of IT, and LESS of you! You don't have to choose between nights out with the girls, and a healthy lifestyle, as long as you're mindful about what you're putting into your body.

We're not saying you can stop exercising, and just drink healthier, but at least this way, you don't have to double up on the workout or have to wake up thinking "what exactly happened last night?" after a long night of overindulgent fun. You CAN have fun, be skinny, and drink! And above all, have fun, enjoy your life, love lots, and be happy!

Cheers to being a Healthy Lush!

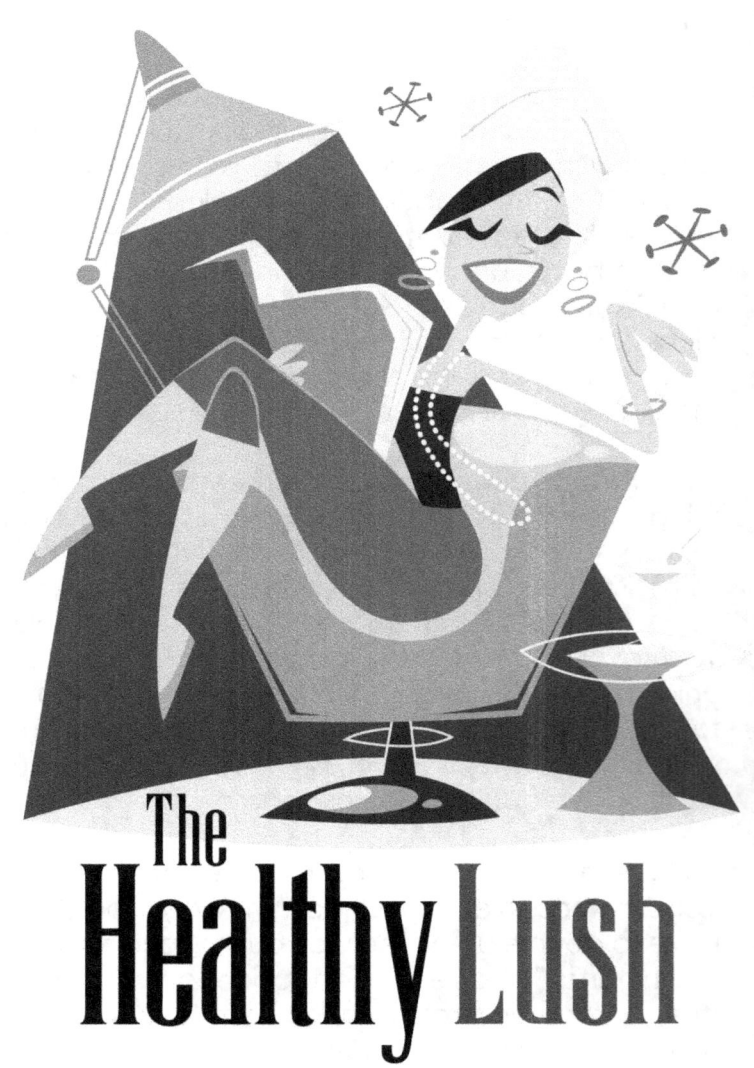

ACKNOWLEDGMENTS

Special thanks to the following people and companies that were essential for completing The Healthy Lush.

Saké Nomi - www.sakenomi.us

E3Live® - www.e3live.com

Mercy® Hangover Prevention Drink
Mercy Nutraceuticals Inc

Navitas Naturals Trail Mix An Organic | Non-GMO Company www.navitasnaturals.com

Q Drinks - www.qdrinks.com

Organic Nation ww.Organicnationspirits.com

Altitude Spirits, Inc www.altitudespirits.com

Square One®
www.squareoneorganicspirits.com

GT's Kombucha™
Millennium Products, Inc
http://www.synergydrinks.com

Zest Kitchen & Bar www.zestslc.com
Salt Lake City, UT.

3 Amigos Tiquela www.3amigostequila.com

Hangover Heaven
www.hangoverheaven.com

*Visit us at **www.TheHealthyLush.com***

REFERENCES

"The Alcohol Debate: Should You or Shouldn't You?"

http://www.medicinenet.com/script/main/art.asp?articlekey=56016 MedicineNet.com

"Alcohol and Nutrition" ~ About.com

http://alcoholism.about.com/cs/alerts/l/blnaa22.htm

"Unhealthy Drinking, Eating Habits Linked" ~ About.com

http://alcoholism.about.com/od/nutrition/a/blniaaa060217.htm

Alcohol: Problems and Solutions
"Healthy Drinking"
"Alcohol, Calories and Weight"
"Facts and Fiction"

http://www2.potsdam.edu/hansondj/HealthIssues/1055517115.html

"Hangover Cures" ~ doublechaser.com

http://www.doublechaser.com/?source=overture

"Alcoholic Beverage Nutrition Facts" ~ Iloveindia.com

http://www.iloveindia.com/nutrition/alcoholic-beverage-facts/index.html

"How Does Alcohol Affect Metabolism"
~ www.metabolic-rate.com

http://www.scribd.com/doc/3039186/How-does-alcohol-affect-metabolism

"Alcohol and Nutrition" ~ healthandgoodness.com

http://www.healthandgoodness.com/nutritiondiet/AlcoholNutrients.htm

"Alcohol Abuse and Nutrition" ~ bacchusnetwork.org

http://www.bacchusgamma.org/alcohol-nutrition.asp

"Nutrition-Healthy Eating (Alcohol)" ~ bbc.co.uk

http://www.bbc.co.uk/health/healthy_living/nutrition/
healthy_alcohol.shtml#what_is_alcohol?

References

"Hangover helper – and tips for healthy drinking"
http://www.goaskalice.columbia.edu/1046.html

"More Americans Drinking Alcohol" ~ ethicsdaily.com
http://www.ethicsdaily.com/article_detail.cfm?AID=1396

"Alcohol – How Drinking Affects Health and Nutrition" ~ doitnow.org
http://www.doitnow.org/pages/120.html

"The Affects of Alcohol on the Body"
"Alcohol and the Body"
"Hangover Cures"
"Standard Drinks" ~ rupissed.com
http://www.rupissed.com/howitworks.html

The Beer Bellie Diet ~ beerbellie.com
http://www.beerbellie.com/Aboutbook.html

How Alcohol Works ~ howstuffworks.com
http://recipes.howstuffworks.com/alcohol2.htm

"Pathways of Alcohol Metabolism" ~ enotalone.com
"The Nutritional Status of Alcoholics"
"The Nutritional Status of Alcoholics: Vitamins"
http://www.enotalone.com/article/11223.html

"Alcohol – it's effects on the body"~ healthchecksystems.com
http://www.healthchecksystems.com/alcohol.htm

"How is alcohol made?"
http://www.at-bristol.org.uk/Alcoholandyou/Facts/howisitmade.html

"Alcohol and Your Body" ~ brown.edu
http://www.brown.edu/Student_Services/Health_Services/
Health_Education/atod/alc_aayb.htm

"Vitamin B12 deficiency" ~ wikipedia.org
http://en.wikipedia.org/wiki/Vitamin_B12_deficiency

The Healthy Lush

"How B Vitamins Work" ~ howstuffworks.com
http://recipes.howstuffworks.com/vitamin-b1.htm

"Fiber- Soluble and Insoluble and Alcohol Sugars"
"Water Facts and Benefits" ~ nutrition.about.com
http://nutrition.about.com/od/askyournutritionist/f/fiberandcarbs.htm

"Journey to making Scotch"
http://running_on_alcohol.tripod.com/id34.html

"Brandy and Cognac" ~ bonappetite.com
http://www.bonappetit.com/tipstools/ingredients/2008/04/brandy_and_cognac

Alcohol and paleo
http://www.paleoplan.com

"Frequently Asked Questions" ~ straightbourbon.com
http://www.straightbourbon.com/faq.html#1

"Dark Rum" ~ Drinksmixer.com
http://www.drinksmixer.com/desc11.html

"About Tequila"
http://www.a1b2c3.com/drugs/alc07.htm

"What is Gin" ~ Foodandbeverageundergound.com
http://www.foodandbeverageunderground.com/origins-of-Gin.html

"How is Rum Made"
http://www.hemingwaysdb.com/rum.php

www.drinkstreet.com
"Drink Beer Get Thin diet"
http://www.realbeer.com/edu/health/beer_diet.php

http://www.realbeer.com/edu/health/calories2.php

"9 Things you Think your Beer says about You" ~ Chris Bucholz
http://www.cracked.com/blog/9-things-you-think-your-beer-says-about-you/

References

"Pros and Cons of Drinking Beer"
http://www.beerandcarbs.com/info.htm

http://www.dumblittleman.com/2008/02/pros-and-cons-of-drinking-beer.html

www.frenchscout.com

"Making of White Wine" ~ wineintro.com

"Making of Red Wine"
http://www.wineintro.com/making/whitewine.html

www.foodandwine.com

Congeners
http://cocktails.about.com/od/cocktailspeak/g/congnr_spk.htm

Types of Drinkers
http://www.alcoholtreatmentclinics.com/types-of-drinkers/

Women and Alcohol Consumption
http://www.nysaes.cornell.edu/fst/faculty/acree/
fs430/notes_thk/03wine&women.html

http://bloodalcoholcalculator.org/

"How Hangovers Work"
www.howstuffworks.com

"How to Avoid a Hangover"
http://www.cocktailtimes.com/awareness/hangover.shtml

"10 Ways to Prevent or Cure a Hangover"
http://itsfood.wordpress.com/2007/04/04/
top-10-ways-to-prevent-or-cure-a-hangover/

"Drinking the Night Away"
http://www.nightworkers.com/drink.html

"Top Ten Hangover Cures"
http://www.forbes.com/2006/12/12/gatorade-excedrin-
tylenol-ent-hr-cx_mf_1212hangover.html

The Healthy Lush

"Top Ten Ways to Prevent a Hangover Cures"
http://itsfood.wordpress.com/2007/04/04/
top-10-ways-to-prevent-or-cure-a-hangover/

"Top Ten Calorie Burning Exercises"
"Swimming and Weight Loss"
http://www.sheknows.com/articles/4774.htm

"You Don't Look So Good" , feature Jane Fonda article
http://www.jane-fonda.net/Feature_2004/Sites/h_aug_c_hangover.htm

"Alcohol Substitutions in Cooking" ~ about.com
http://mideastfood.about.com/od/tipsandtechniques/a/alcohol_subs.htm

"Allergy to Wine" ~ allergynotes.blogsmot.com
http://allergynotes.blogspot.com/2008/09/allergy-to-wine-correct-diagnosis-may.html

"Learn all about Resveratrol"
http://www.nutritional-supplement-guides.com/Resveratrol.html

http://www.Rupissed.com/hangover cures

References

- **Nutrition for Dummies (book)**
- **The Skinny Bitch (book)**
- **The China Study (book)**
- **The Drunken Botanist (book)**
- **The South Beach Diet (book)**
- **Nature's Cures (book)**
- **Physical Activity and Health (book)**
- **The Body Code (book)**
- **How's Your Drink (book)**
- **Will Mix for Sex (book)**
- **Naturally Thin (book)**
- **Controlling Your Drinking (book)**
- **Eat This, Not That (book)**
- **The Little Black Book of Cocktails (book)**
- **Eat 4 Your Type (book)**